THE IMPACT OF A UNIQUE COOPERATIVE AMERICAN UNIVERSITY USAID FUNDED SPEECH-LANGUAGE PATHOLOGIST, AUDIOLOGIST, AND DEAF EDUCATOR B.S. DEGREE PROGRAM IN THE GAZA STRIP

Front cover:
Photograph taken in President Arafat's office in Gaza City,1994, showing the author, Dr. Franklin H. Silverman (left), Dr. Hatem Abu Ghazaheh, Chairman, Society for the Care of the Handicapped in the Gaza Strip (center), and President Yassar Arafat.

THE IMPACT OF A UNIQUE COOPERATIVE AMERICAN UNIVERSITY USAID FUNDED SPEECH-LANGUAGE PATHOLOGIST, AUDIOLOGIST, AND DEAF EDUCATOR B.S. DEGREE PROGRAM IN THE GAZA STRIP

Franklin H. Silverman
and
Robert Moulton

Mellen Studies in Education
Volume 67

The Edwin Mellen Press
Lewiston•Queenston•Lampeter

MW

Library of Congress Cataloging-in-Publication Data

Silverman, Franklin H., 1933-
The impact of a unique cooperative American university, USAID funded speech-language pathologist, audiologist, and deaf educator B.S. degree program in the Gaza Strip / Franklin H. Silverman, Robert D. Moulton.
p. cm. -- (Mellen studies in education ; v. 67)
Includes bibliographical references and index.
ISBN 0-7734-7189-8
1. Speech therapy--Study and teaching--Gaza Strip. 2. Speech therapists--Training of--Gaza Strip. I. Moulton, Robert D. II. Title. III. Series.

RC428.5 .S545 2002
616.85'5'00711531--dc21

2001052157

This is volume 67 in the continuing series
Mellen Studies in Education
Volume 67 ISBN 0-7734-7189-8
MSE Series ISBN 0-88946-935-0

A CIP catalog record for this book is available from the British Library.

The Edwin Mellen Press
Box 450
Lewiston, New York
USA 14092-0450

The Edwin Mellen Press
Box 67
Queenston, Ontario
CANADA L0S 1L0

The Edwin Mellen Press, Ltd.
Lampeter, Ceredigion, Wales
UNITED KINGDOM SA48 8LT

Printed in the United States of America

3/26/07

To our Palestinian students, whose dedication and professionalism contributed greatly to the success of this project

Table of Contents

Preface

This book describes a unique B.S. degree training program that was conducted jointly by a state university (Lamar University in Beaumont, Texas) and a private Jesuit university (Marquette University in Milwaukee, Wisconsin) in the Gaza Strip between 1992 and 1996 and its impacts on the participants and others. Faculty from both universities traveled to the Gaza Strip and taught courses while living there. The project, which was funded by a ten million dollar grant from the United States Agency for International Development (USAID), resulted in both the creation of state-of-the-art facilities in the Gaza Strip for providing clinical services to speech and hearing handicapped children and adults and in the training of 33 Palestinian young men and women (most of whom were residents of refugee camps) as speech-language pathologists, audiologists, and teachers of the deaf. Their training closely approximated that for these professions in the United States.

This book contains information that is likely to be of interest to scholars and practitioners in several fields. It would perhaps be of greatest interest to ones in the field of higher education because it provides a model that could be used to develop programs for training other kinds of professionals, in other developing countries. Our experience would make it unnecessary for those who do so to have to completely "reinvent the wheel." It also contains information that would be of interest to scholars who are researching the Gaza Strip and/or the relationship between the United States and the Palestinian Authority. Furthermore, the book contains information that would be of interest to those studying the impacts of projects funded by USAID. And, of course, there is information that would be of interest to scholars and practitioners in speech-language pathology, audiology, deaf education, and other rehabilitation-related fields, particularly those in developing countries.

It isn't possible to give credit to the many sources from which the ideas in this book have been drawn. This book is the result of almost 10 years of involvement with this project and its aftermath, as well as hundreds of hours of conversations with our students and other residents of the Gaza Strip. Thus, we cannot credit this or that idea to a specific person, but we can say "thank you" to all whose ideas we have borrowed.

Franklin H. Silverman, Ph.D.
Robert Moulton, Ph.D.

Foreword

While the establishment by Marquette University in the Gaza Strip of a bachelor degree program in communicative disorders was at some levels a project unlike any ever tackled by this institution, it turned out to be a uniquely valuable effort, one that fit well indeed with our mission as a Catholic and Jesuit university of fostering excellence, faith, leadership, and service, especially the service of those in greatest and most pressing need.

When this new academic enterprise was first being discussed, I was then serving as chair of our Board's Academic Affairs Committee. After listening to a briefing on the plan proposed by the project team, the committee's first reaction was, "Gaza? Can we really accomplish such an ambitious project under the conditions people face in the Gaza Strip?" But when we considered the eager willingness of a number of Marquette professors to get involved in this effort and the confidence that the university's administration had in what Dr. Franklin Silverman of Marquette and Dr. Robert Moulton of Lamar University had proposed, we were happy to give it our support. Nevertheless, it remained a complex undertaking, a real challenge to pull off successfully, and so I am pleased that its leaders have decided to present to the wider academic community a detailed description of what they were able to accomplish and of what it took to achieve those results. Theirs in a good story to tell, one that is not theirs alone but that of many others as well, not least a number of local leaders in Gaza itself who worked closely with the American team to ensure a successful outcome for the project.

As you will read in the pages that follow, through this one-time program Marquette University was able to offer a bachelor of science degree in speech pathology, audiology, and deaf education to thirty-three young men and women in

Gaza. The students who completed it, most of whom were residents of refugee camps, were thereby empowered to gain access to a brighter future than they might otherwise achieved without this educational advantage. Even more importantly, the training they received has enabled them to provide competent professional assistance to thousands of handicapped children in one of the most impoverished places on earth.

There are many ways in which this project was unique:

- None of the students were Catholic. Of the thirty-three students in the program thirty-one were Moslem and two were Protestant.
- None of the courses for the degree were taken on Marquette's campus in Milwaukee. Marquette faculty and others who taught in the program traveled to the Gaza Strip to teach their courses. They did this mainly because it would be better in the end to train these students in the very cultural environment in which they would continue to live and work.
- In offering this program, Marquette worked in close cooperation with a public university in Texas, Lamar University, and a non-government organization based in Gaza, the Society for the Care of the Handicapped. This collaborative effort proved very beneficial for all concerned.
- Marquette did not benefit financially from the program. The university received less than half the amount of tuition per credit hour than it would have for a program on its main campus. The revenue received did not even cover the salaries of participating faculty and the other direct expenses incurred.

Following the values stressed by the founder of the Jesuits, St. Ignatius of Loyola, Jesuit education seeks to encourage and empower students to become "men and women for others," men and women, that is, who believe it essential to look beyond their own self-interest and their own needs to those of others, especially the poor and marginalized in our world. The graduates of Marquette's Gaza program have demonstrated ample willingness to do so, particularly through their clear commitment to helping handicapped children.

In short, we at Marquette are proud of having contributed significantly to the success of this project. Just as the students in Gaza who earned Marquette degrees benefited from the experience, so we as an institution have also benefited in a number of tangible and intangible ways. On the basis of our own experience I can in good conscious recommend that other colleges and universities in the United States and other developed nations give serious consideration to entering into partnering relationships of this sort. The practical information that Drs. Silverman and Moulton share here with readers should provide very useful information that can help to guide others interested in undertaking this type of project in a Third World environment.

Robert A. Wild, S.J.

President

Marquette University

Chapter 1
The Need

Communication is the one activity we engage in that no other animal appears to be capable of doing better. That is, there is at least one animal that clearly exceeds our sensory and/or motor abilities to do each of the other tasks we're capable of doing (e.g., hearing, seeing, and running). Our ability to communicate in a sophisticated manner about the past and future as well as the present has been responsible, in large part, for our being able to develop technologically and otherwise to the extent we have.

There are few activities you engage in that don't require you to communicate with others. Consider the following scenario: When you awake tomorrow morning, you find yourself completely unable to talk well enough to be understood. You're able to hear and understand speech as well as ever and your ability to think and reason is unimpaired. But when you try to talk, your tongue won't move. It just lies still, paralyzed on the floor of your mouth. A physician examines you and concludes that the paralysis is due to damage to the nerves that innervate the tongue musculature and that their condition is unlikely to improve. What impacts do you think not being able to talk normally would have on your life? Would you be able to do the same work? In what ways would it affect your plans for the future? How would it affect your social and family life? How would it affect how you feel about yourself? There are many other scenarios (such as sudden-onset hearing loss) that could illustrate our dependence on our ability to communicate.

If you are like most persons, you probably will have difficulty answering these questions because you take being able to talk and hear for granted (as you do being able to walk and to use your hands). This is not particularly surprising because you've been able to do both for as long as you can remember. Babies begin paying attention to sound and using their voices to communicate within a few minutes after being born. For example, they cry to tell us that they are uncomfortable and they stop crying to indicate that all is right with their world. Only persons who have had difficulty communicating, either temporarily or permanently, can fully appreciate the impacts it can have on almost all aspects of living. Some of these impacts will be described in the next section.

HANDICAPS CAUSED BY SPEECH, LANGUAGE, AND HEARING DISORDERS

Being unable to hear and/or speak normally can handicap a child or adult by doing one or more of the following:

- Interfering with communication
- Calling adverse attention to the person
- Causing the person to have a poor self-image

Some implications of each are dealt with in this section.

Interfering with Communication

A speech, language, or hearing disorder can impede the transmission of information between speaker and listener in several ways. First, it can interfere with receiving information. Being deaf , for example, can make it difficult or impossible for a person to understand through hearing what people say.

A speech, hearing, or language disorder also can interfere in a number of ways with a speaker's ability to transmit information to a listener. One way, for example, would be by preventing a speaker from finding (remembering) some of the words (particularly nouns) that he or she needs to communicate messages. It could also prevent a speaker from fully controlling the musculature of the speech mechanism (for example, that of her tongue), thereby reducing the *intelligibility* (understandability) of what he or she says.

Calling Adverse Attention to the Person

Just as there are negative stereotypes for members of certain racial and religious groups, there are also preconceived notions about persons who have certain speech, language, and/or hearing disorders. These include being deaf or hard-of-hearing, being unable to speak, stuttering, and lisping. If you expect a person to have certain personality characteristics or to behave in a certain undesirable way because he or she has a particular disorder, your expectation can cause you to perceive the person as having these characteristics and exhibiting these behaviors (Johnson, 1946).

Causing the Person to Have a Poor Self-Image

Having abnormal speech, language, or hearing can influence your self-concept. It can make you dislike yourself, which can cause you to be one or more of the following: unhappy, depressed, overly sensitive, frustrated, suicidal, embarrassed, pessimistic, emotionally unstable, defensive, introverted, frightened, or tense. Liking yourself is a necessary condition for developing and maintaining productive, enjoyable relationships with others.

For further information about either speech, language, or hearing disorders and how having one can cause a person to be handicapped, see Silverman (1995).

THE GAZA STRIP

The B.S. degree program that is the focus of this book was designed to train communicative disorders specialists for employment in the Gaza Strip. It was conducted between 1992 and 1996 in the city of Gaza in the Gaza Strip (the preferred Palestinian term for it is the Gaza District). The Gaza Strip is a narrow strip of coastline (about 40 km) on the Mediterranean Sea that is bordered to the south by Egypt and to the North and East by Israel. Its width at its minimum is 6 km and at its maximum is 14 km. It has an area of about 363 sq. km (140 sq. miles). The largest city is Gaza (from which the strip got its name). More than 98 percent of the city's population were Arabic-speaking Moslems (Turner, 1999). The rest were mostly Christians.

The Arab population of the Gaza Strip during the period that we conducted our program was probably between 750,000 and 800,000 (Turner, 1999). Approximately 40 percent were indigenous and the rest were refugees. There was also an Israeli population of between 4,000 and 5,000. The percentage of the Arab population of preschool or school age was very high because the fertility rate of the women there (i.e., 8.8 children per family) has been the highest in the world (Turner, 1999).

Palestinian refugee families resided in one of eight camps: Jabalia, al-Shatti, Nuseirt, al-Boureij, Dir al-Balah, Meghazi, Khan Yunis, and Rafah. More than half of our students resided in one of the camps. Some families had lived in these camps since shortly after the Arab-Israeli War in 1948. The camps were administered and funded by the United Nations Relief and Works Agency (UNRWA). The poverty level within the camps was very high, and living conditions, at best, were marginal (see Daughty & El Aydi, 1995; Davies & Johnson, 1991; Frankel, 1996; Hass, 1999; Qleibo, 1992; Roy, 1995).

The city of Gaza is more than 3,000 years old. Anciently, Gaza was the residence of the Egyptian Governor to Canaan. In the 13th century BC, the Philistines arrived and, according to the bible, Gaza is where Sampson was imprisoned after Delilah made him weak by cutting off his hair.

The Gaza Strip came under Moslem rule in the 7th century AD. It was occupied by England between 1922 and 1948 (see Segev, 2000), by Egypt during most of the period from 1948 and 1967, and by Israel from 1967 (after the Six-Day War) to 1994. In 1994, as a result of the signing of the Oslo Agreement, most of the Israeli occupying troops left and control was passed on to the Palestinian National Authority, which still held it when this chapter was written. For further historical information about the Gaza Strip, see Butt (1995).

SPEECH, LANGUAGE, AND HEARING DISORDERS AMONG RESIDENTS OF THE GAZA STRIP

The information available about the prevalence of speech, language, and hearing disorders among the residents of the Gaza Strip in the late 1980s and early 1990s was in large part anecdotal or inferential. Nevertheless, the available information on the extent of communication disorders and the lack of treatment services within the Gaza Strip was sufficient to convince the United States Agency for International Development (USAID) to fund our project at 10 million dollars (U.S.).

Dr. Hatem Abu Ghazaleh, a British-trained physician who was co-director of the Project and Chairman of the Society for the Care of the Handicapped in the Gaza Strip, conducted a needs study in 1990. He estimated that of the 250,000 school-age children in the Gaza Strip, 20,000 to 30,000 had hearing, speech, and/or language disorders sufficiently severe to disable and/or handicap them. His data indicated that almost none of them had received any speech-language pathology, audiology, and/or deaf education services. He estimated that least 2,000 of these children had some degree of hearing loss and 500 to 750 of them were deaf. Furthermore, Dr. Ghazaleh concluded that there were at least as many adults in the Gaza Strip who had speech, language, and/or hearing disorders severe enough to disable and/or handicap them and almost none had received any rehabilitation or educational services. Our experiences in Gaza between 1992 and 1996 have caused us to conclude that Dr. Abu Ghazaleh's prevelance estimates were conservative, particularly the one for the number of persons in the Strip who are deaf.

The percentages of the persons in the Gaza Strip who appeared to have speech, language, and/or hearing disorders were high by western standards. The factors responsible for it being so high probably included the following:

- Poor nutrition and health care
- Head injuries suffered during the military occupation and intifada
- Consanguine marriages

Some examples of how each undoubtedly contributed the relatively high prevalence of speech, language, and/or hearing disorders in the Gaza Strip during the early- and mid-1990s are given below.

Poor Nutrition and Health Care

The health care that most residents of the Gaza Strip received during this period was relatively poor for two reasons—poverty and lack of availability. Unemployment exceeded 50 percent for men and was close to 100 percent for women. Most of these who had jobs (in either Gaza or Israel) received very low salaries. Even residents who could afford to pay for health care services often couldn't get them because they weren't available.

There are at least two ways that poor health care and/or nutrition could have contributed to the relatively high rate of speech, language, and hearing disorders. One would be a lack of adequate nutrition and prenatal services during pregnancy increasing the prevalence of congenital disorders, such as cleft palate, deafness, and mental deficiency. And the second would be pathological conditions of the speech and hearing mechanisms (e.g., middle ear infections) not being ameliorated soon enough to keep these mechanisms from being damaged.

Head Injuries Suffered During the Military Occupation and Intifada

The Gaza Strip was under Israeli military occupation between 1967 and 1994. This occupation was opposed by almost all of the Arab inhabitants and culminated in the uprising (i.e., gorilla warfare) from 1987 to 1993 referred to as the Intifada. Guns were fired, rocks were thrown, and many belligerents and innocent bystanders (including young children) received head injuries that affected their hearing, speech, and/or language abilities.

Consanguine Marriages

A number of factors—including high population density, large extended families, strict rules regarding male-female contact, and arranged marriages—have resulted in a considerable degree of intermarriage in the Gaza Strip (Brown, Abu Ghazaleh, & Neufeldt, 1996). It was reported, for example, that more than 50 percent of marriages were between first cousins (Saunders, 1985). This would be expected to result in a higher than usual incidence of the recessive genetic conditions that tend to be associated with speech, language, and/or hearing disorders, such as cleft palate and deafness.

FACILITIES AND PERSONNEL AVAILABLE PRIOR TO THE BEGINNING OF THIS PROJECT FOR TREATING AND EDUCATING PERSONS IN THE GAZA STRIP WHO WERE SPEECH, LANGUAGE, AND/OR HEARING IMPAIRED

Prior to the beginning of this project, there were no audiologists or facilities in the Gaza Strip for testing hearing and fitting hearing aids. Nor were there any speech-language pathologists or facilities for treating persons who had a speech or language disorder. The few residents who had received such services had done so in Israel or in some other country.

DR. HATEM ABU GHAZALEH AND THE SOCIETY FOR THE CARE OF THE HANDICAPPED IN THE GAZA STRIP

A beginning had already been made in the Gaza Strip in developing special education and rehabilitation services and training special education and rehabilitation professionals to provide them. The person who had been primarily responsible for planning and implementing these services and training programs was Dr. Hatem Abu Ghazaleh, the co-director of our project. Our project was, in fact, a component of Dr. Ghazaleh's attempt to develop special education and rehabilitation services in the Gaza Strip that were comparable to those in western countries (see Brown, Abu Ghazaleh, & Neufeldt, 1996) .

Dr. Hatem Abu Ghazaleh

Dr. Hatem Abu Ghazaleh was responsible, directly or indirectly, for almost all of the other special education and rehabilitation programs in the Gaza Strip from the mid-1970s to the mid-1990s. Those that he didn't initiate were at least partially staffed by persons that he had a hand in training. Dr. Ghazaleh was born in Jerusalem in 1935. He received his primary education in Jerusalem and his secondary schooling in Gaza. His university education and his medical training occurred in England where he graduated from King's College, Cambridge, and the Westminster Hospital, in London. For a fifteen year period beginning in 1960, he practiced as a general surgeon in Gaza. Since 1975 when he became aware of the lack of special education and rehabilitation services in the Gaza Strip, he has abandoned his surgical practice and devoted all of his time and family resources to the handicapped children living there. Because Dr. Ghazaleh believed that handicapped children in Gaza deserved education and rehabilitation services on a par with those available in industrialized nations, he enlisted the aid of special education and rehabilitation leaders from universities in the United States and Canada and partnered with their institutions to initiate programs to train Palestinian professionals in the Gaza Strip. The institutions with which he partnered included the University of Calgary in Canada and Lamar University and Marquette University in United States.

The Society for the Care of the Handicapped in the Gaza Strip

The organization that Dr. Ghazaleh founded in 1975 to advocate for and attempt to meet the special education and rehabilitation needs of handicapped children and adults was the Society for the Care of the Handicapped in the Gaza Strip. This Society, of which Dr. Ghazaleh was Chairman, was governed by a seven member Board of Directors that made fundamental policy and programmatic decisions. In 1994, the Society employed a staff of about 330 and provided services to about 5,000 persons, mostly children. Its administrative offices and some of its services were housed in the Sun Day Care Center building in the suburb of Gaza called Rimal.

The aims of the Society during the period of our project (i.e., 1992 to 1996) included the following:

1. Advance social consciousness of the problem of mental retardation and the understanding of its nature and its various aspects in the hope of modifying attitudes toward all handicaps.

2. Establish centers for the care and rehabilitation of the handicapped throughout the Gaza Strip, including high quality vocational training programs.

3. Establish units for handicapped children in mainstream educational institutions.

4. Provide a service to the homes of handicapped and non-handicapped infants and young children to train the mothers and help the families cope as early as possible.

5. Establish high quality training programs to produce Arabic-speaking experts in the fields of special education and rehabilitation.

6. Advance research and conduct surveys on the incidence and type of various handicaps in the Gaza Strip in comparison with world figures.

The Society provided six major services other than those specifically for persons who are speech or hearing impaired: the Sun Day Care Center (for mentally retarded children); the Mother's Home Care/Early Intervention Program; a home-based early intervention program to teach the mothers of non-handicapped children at risk of developmental delay because of the prevailing adverse environmental conditions; the Fahd El Lababidi Center for Special Education; a vocational training and rehabilitation service; and a teacher and rehabilitation specialist training program.

Chapter 2
The Plan

In 1991, a group of speech and hearing consultants from the United States and Jordan visited Gaza and conducted a feasibility study. These professionals (several of whom were from Lamar University) recommended that the Society for the Care of the Handicapped in the Gaza Strip establish a personnel training program, a speech and hearing clinic, and a home-based service delivery program. Based on these recommendations, the Society did the following:

- Partnered with Lamar University to establish a personnel training program in Gaza. From an initial group of over 200 applicants, a group of 33 Palestinian college-age students were selected to become speech-language pathologists, audiologists, and teachers of the deaf. Short- and long-term professors from the U.S. were recruited for teaching the speech-, hearing-, and language-related courses and training of the 33 students began in Gaza in 1992. In 1994, the Society and Lamar University partnered with Marquette University to provide the 18 course liberal arts component for the program and award a B.S. degree.
- Constructed and equipped a state-of-the-art audiology clinic (including a laboratory for making earmolds and repairing hearing aids) in Gaza that offered hearing testing and the following hearing aid services: testing, fitting, repair, and the production of earmolds. The clinic became fully operational in 1993. A state-of-the-art clinic for the diagnosis and treatment of speech and language disorders was constructed the next year. Both clinics were used for providing students with supervised

practicum experience and for providing clinical services to the men, women, and children of the Gaza Strip.

- Began delivering services to Palestinians with speech, language, and/or hearing disorders. These services were provided through the new audiology clinic (beginning in 1993), the new speech-language pathology clinic (beginning in 1994), and the mothers' home training program. The Society had used the mothers' program for many years to meet the educational and rehabilitation needs of thousands of other handicapped or at-risk children: This program took teachers and therapists into the homes of handicapped children to both train mothers to provide at least some of the educational and/or rehabilitative services their children required and to supervise the mothers as they provided these services to their children.

Some of the issues that were considered and tasks that were done while planning for carrying out these recommendations are indicated here.

DECIDING HOW TO MEET THE NEED

There were four options considered for beginning to meet the educational and rehabilitation needs of persons residing in Gaza who had speech, language, and/or hearing disorders: hiring professionals from elsewhere; training teachers, psychologists, or physicians in Gaza to provide these educational and rehabilitation services; training persons to provide services at a paraprofessional ("technician") level; and/or training persons to provide them at a professional level. The practicality and potential advantages and disadvantages of each option will be considered here.

The first option—*hiring professionals from elsewhere*—would enable educational and rehabilitation services for persons who had speech, language, and/or hearing disorders to be offered sooner than would any of the other three options. And it would also result in the services being provided by fully-trained professionals. In the past, this option has been utilized as a first step to providing such services in several Arab countries, including the Kingdom of Saudi Arabia.*

---

*There is a communicative disorders training program at King Saud University in Riyadh, Kingdom of Saudi Arabia.

One of the main limitations of this option as a long-term solution is finding a sufficient number of professionals who speak the national language(s) and are both familiar and comfortable with the country's culture. While it certainly is possible to offer educational and rehabilitation services in a country without being able to speak its national language(s) by using interpreters, doing so can lead to misunderstandings, particularly when professionals are not familiar with the prevailing culture. Another major limitation of this option is financial. Foreign professionals almost always have to be paid relatively high salaries to attract them (unless, of course, they're volunteers—e.g., members of the Peace Corps), and few developing countries are likely to have the funds to hire enough foreign professionals to meet their needs long-term.

The second option—*training other local professionals to provide these services*—probably would enable services to be offered sooner than either the third or fourth option plus be less expensive to implement than either of them. Both of us have provided such training (through continuing education workshops) to healthcare and special education professionals in developing countries.

One limitation of this option as a long-term solution is finding a sufficient number of local professionals who would have the time to provide these services. In most developing countries, there are too few healthcare and special education professionals to even come close to meeting the need for the services that they are licensed to provide. A second limitation of this option—perhaps the major one—is that those providing the services would not be fully trained to do so. They, of course, could be helpful to some degree, but probably not to the maximum extent possible.

The third option—*training personnel at a paraprofessional level*—would be less expensive and time-consuming than the fourth option and would be likely to yield a higher quality of services than the second. Those completing such a training program would probably receive a certificate rather than a bachelor's or a master's degree. This option was, in fact, utilized in some developed countries when they began offering rehabilitation services. It is also an aspect of the community based rehabilitation philosophy.

The main limitation of this option as a long-term solution is that the level of the services yielded by its adoption is unlikely to be as high as those yielded by the fourth one, particularly if there aren't sufficient fully-trained professionals to supervise the paraprofessional ones. Consequently, the rehabilitation and special education services available in a country that adopts this option (particularly if supervision isn't adequate) are unlikely to be of as high in quality as those available in developed countries.

The fourth option—*training personnel at a professional level*—is the most costly and time-consuming. The training provided would have to be equivalent to that in the United States, Canada, and other developed countries and those trained would have to receive at least a bachelor's degree for successfully completing it. However, adopting this option would probably result in higher quality services being available than would adoption of one of the others.

Dr. Ghazaleh (the Director of the Society for the Care of the Handicapped in the Gaza Strip) decided to adopt the fourth option for the speech-language pathologist, audiologist, and deaf educator training programs. He wanted the rehabilitation and special educational services available in Gaza to be as close as possible to those available in developed countries. Consequently, the curriculums followed for the training programs in Gaza were based, in large part, on the training recommendations of the U.S.-based American Speech-Language-Hearing Association, which governs institutions that train audiologists and speech-language pathologists, and of the Council on Education of the Deaf, which governs the training of teachers of deaf children in the United States.

The first option—hiring professionals from elsewhere—was also adopted for this project, though indirectly. The ASHA-certified speech-language pathologists and audiologists who supervised clinical practicum in Gaza and the deaf education specialists who directed student teaching there did provide direct services as they demonstrated best practices.

DECIDING WHETHER TO TRAIN PERSONNEL IN GAZA OR ELSEWHERE

After adopting the fourth option, the next decision that we had to make was where to do the training. The two options we considered were doing it in Gaza or in the United States. We decided to do it in Gaza for the following reasons:

- We wanted to maximize the odds that the graduates of our program would remain in Gaza.
- We wanted their practicum experience to be in their culture.

- We wanted to be able to begin helping persons in Gaza who were communicatively impaired as quickly as possible.
- The ability of some (perhaps most) of our students to understand, speak, read, and write English wasn't adequate for admission to a university in the United States.

Some of the ways that each of these impacted on our decision are indicated below.

Our primary goal was to provide clinical services to communicatively handicapped persons who lived in the Gaza Strip. It would, of course, be necessary for the graduates of our program to remain in Gaza to achieve this goal. We believed that they would be more likely to do so if they were trained there because a relatively high percentage of the students from developing countries who come to the United States for an education never return.

If our plan was successful and our students remained in Gaza after graduating, the language/culture of their clients would be Arabic. Consequently, it would be more sensible for our students to have their clinical practicum experience in Gaza than in the United States.

We wanted to begin providing clinical services in Gaza as soon as possible. This goal could obviously be achieved more rapidly by having the students do their practicum in Gaza, supervised by fully-qualified professionals who could also provide such services.

The final consideration was our students' abilities to understand, speak, read, and write English. For the majority of our students, English proficiency at the beginning of the training program was low and they would not have been able to compete successfully at universities in the United States. For this project, we began with a large group of perspective students, selected those with the better English skills, and then provided English as a Second Language (ESL) training throughout the entire five year training period.

DEFINING GRADUATES' SCOPE OF PRACTICE

One of the first steps in creating a professional training program is to specify at least some of the services that will define the *scope of practice* of its graduates. The scope of practice for our graduates in speech-language pathology and audiology was to be that of persons who had a Certificate of Clinical Competence in one of these specialties from the American Speech-Language-Hearing Association.

And the scope of practice for our graduates in deaf education is that of teachers of the deaf in the United States.

PARTNERING

If all of the resources needed to conduct a professional training program are not available locally, one option for securing the ones that aren't is for the local entity to partner with one or more "foreign" ones. This option was utilized here. The Society for the Care of the Handicapped in the Gaza Strip (SCHGS) had to secure the following resources to implement this training program:

- Planning for curriculum and facilities
- Funding
- Faculty
- Facilities and equipment for providing practicum experience
- Cooperation from Israel and from the Palestinian Authority

The partnering relationships that were developed for providing these resources are described below.

The SCHGS initiated planning for the program by partnering with Lamar University in Beaumont, Texas, USA. Lamar is a state-supported university. One of us (RM) was Associate Vice President for Research and Graduate Dean there at that time. RM collaborated with the SCHGS on planning curriculum, identifying facility and equipment needs, and preparing a grant application to fund the project. With Dr. Ghazaleh, RM served as the co-director of the training program. Lamar University provided faculty for some of the audiology, deaf education, and speech-language pathology courses.

The funding partner for the project was the United States Agency for International Development (USAID). The grantee was the SCHGS rather than the Palestinian Authority (which didn't exist when the grant was funded). Toward the end of the project , USAID did, however, divert some money from the grant to the Palestinian Authority for other purposes (e.g., paying the salaries of its police).

Marquette University in Milwaukee, Wisconsin, USA was the other University with which the SCHGS partnered. It is both private and Catholic (Jesuit). Marquette University provided faculty for some of the speech-language pathology courses, all of the liberal arts courses, and awarded Bachelor of Science degrees to the 33 graduates of the program.

In addition to these three formal partnerships, there were two informal ones. One was with the Israelis who were governing Gaza prior to May, 1994. Some cooperation, for example, had to be secured from them (possibly just "looking the other way") to enable the facilities for the audiology and speech-language pathology clinics to be constructed. The other was with the Palestinian Authority after it assumed control in Gaza. The Palestinian Authority, for example, facilitated securing a telephone line for the speech clinic.

DEVELOPING A CURRICULUM

The professional curriculum for the speech-language pathology and audiology components of the training program closely approximated those required for the Certificates of Clinical Competence in Speech-Language Pathology and Audiology from the American Speech-Language-Hearing Association. And that for its deaf education component closely approximated the requirements for a major in deaf education at Lamar University. The curriculum for the liberal arts component of the program was based on that required by the Department of Speech Pathology and Audiology at Marquette University for a Bachelor of Science degree. All of the courses are listed and described in Appendix B.

PLANNING FACILITIES

The facilities that were needed to implement the program included the following: classrooms, housing for short-term faculty, an audiology clinic (including an ear-mold laboratory), and a speech clinic. The first two–classrooms and housing–already existed. They had been acquired (i.e., built or leased) for training programs that the SCHGS had conducted previously. No facilities existed in the Gaza Strip that were appropriate for an audiology or speech-language clinic. Therefore, state-of-the-art physical facilities were designed and built for the project. Local craftsmen and materials were used.

DETERMINING EQUIPMENT AND SUPPLY NEEDS

A considerable amount of equipment and supplies were needed, particularly for the audiology and speech clinics. The equipment ranged from photocopy machines and computers to hearing-testing booths and sophisticated audiometers. The types needed and their cost had to be estimated for the grant application.

ESTIMATING PERSONNEL COSTS

These included salaries and overhead-related expenses for both long- and short-term faculty and support staff. They also included travel expenses and "room and board" for short-term faculty.

SECURING ISRAELI AND PALESTINIAN AUTHORITY SUPPORT

Because the Gaza Strip was occupied and governed by the Israeli Defense Force (IDF) when the project was being planned, some support from the Israelis was essential. This support was secured. One reason probably was Dr. Ghazaleh being respected for his humanitarian work by at least some of the leadership of the IDF in Gaza. Another probably was the project being supported by USAID, an agency from which the government of Israel received millions of dollars annually.

After the Palestinian Authority assumed control in Gaza, its support for the project was regarded as being essential. President Arafat was informed about the project, met several times with some of its U. S. faculty, and even agreed to be the speaker at the graduation. His personal intervention, for example, resulted in our being able to get a telephone line for the speech clinic even though there was a long waiting list for one.

LOBBYING FOR UNITED STATES GOVERNMENT SUPPORT

Dr. Ghazaleh had spent considerable time in Washington lobbying for support for SCHGS projects. On the wall of his office there was a photograph of him with President Bush and one of him with Senator Ted Kennedy. He kept a furnished apartment in Virginia, very close to Washington, D.C. and convenient for his frequent lobbying trips.

PREPARING THE PROPOSAL FOR SECURING FUNDING

The grant applications for the project were drafted by one of us (RM) in collaboration with Dr. Ghazaleh and submitted to USAID in behalf of the Society for the Care of the Handicapped in the Gaza Strip. The Society had previously received major funding from USAID for smaller personnel training projects, those dealing with training special education teachers. In 1991, USAID provided the Society with start-up funding for speech and hearing programs, including the construction of the audiology clinic. And in the summer of 1993, USAID awarded the Society a three-year, 10.4 million dollar grant to support the communicative disorders training program.

The budget sections in the USAID grant applications did not specifically mention funding for the liberal arts component of the bachelor's degree program. Lamar University, like most state-supported universities at that time (which was before Internet-based distance learning became popular), couldn't award a bachelor's degree to somebody who wasn't a resident of the institution's home state and had never attended classes on its campus. It could, however, award such persons a certificate for successfully completing a prescribed program of professional study. Since the objective of the project was to train speech and hearing professionals and having the liberal arts component of a bachelor's degree wasn't essential for doing so, it was initially argued that the training program could accomplish its objective by awarding a certificate of program completion rather than a bachelors degree at the end of the training program. And the members of the panel who reviewed the grant application for USAID apparently agreed.

Dr. Ghazaleh had wanted the training program to culminate in a bachelor's degree and made a few unsuccessful attempts prior to 1994 to interest a private university in partnering with the Society and Lamar by providing the liberal arts component for the bachelor's degree and awarding it. One university that he contacted apparently did exhibit some interest in pursuing such a partnership, but the amount that it would charge for tuition and indirect costs considerably exceeded that which could be made available for the purpose from the existing USAID grants.

During the spring and/or summer of 1994, many of the students finally understood that at the end of the program they would be receiving a certificate rather than a university degree, even though they were told this on the first day and frequently thereafter. They appeared to be quite disturbed by this—they really wanted a bachelor's degree, probably (at least in part) because they regarded it as a "ticket" to a good job. During the summer of 1994, one of the authors (FHS) who is on the faculty of a private Jesuit university (Marquette University) was in Gaza teaching a clinical course. Because of the high level of interest among the students in receiving a bachelor's degree and Dr. Ghazaleh's own interest in their doing so, Dr. Ghazaleh asked FHS to determine when he returned to Milwaukee whether Marquette would have any interest in pursuing the possibility of partnering with the Society and Lamar by providing the liberal arts component and awarding the students a bachelor's degree. In September 1994, FHS met with Dr. Francis Lazarus, who at that time was Marquette's Vice President for Academic Affairs. Dr. Lazarus became a strong advocate for Marquette's involvement with the project and it was primarily because of his extraordinary efforts, farsightedness, and creativity that Marquette's involvement with it became a reality.

In October, 1994, Marquette University offered to partner with the Society and Lamar University by offering in Gaza 18 core courses in the liberal arts. The Training Agreement stated that students who successfully completed these core courses and the intensive training from Lamar University would satisfy the Marquette University academic requirements for a Bachelor of Science degree in Communication Disorders. It further stated that the budget would not include indirect costs and would only call for a payment of $169,170 for tuition for the 18 courses and fees. This was $657,588 less than the 33 students would have paid if they had taken these courses on the Marquette campus. Airline tickets for Marquette faculty to and from Gaza were to be provided by the Society.

As we've indicated previously, funding for the liberal arts courses and for degree- and travel-related costs had not been budgeted for in the three year USAID grant. The funding for costs associated with the bachelor's degree came from a $1,000 fee paid by each of the students (or their immediate or extended families) and a reallocating of funds from the grant.

RECRUITING FACULTY

The recruitment of U.S. faculty and staff for the Project, though successful, turned out to be considerably more difficult than anticipated. One of us (RM) was responsible for recruiting faculty to teach speech-language pathology, audiology, and deaf education courses and to staff the audiology and speech-language pathology clinics. And Dr. Francis Lazarus (Marquette's V.P. for Academic Affairs) was responsible for recruiting faculty to teach the 18 liberal arts courses.

Two of the reasons why it was more difficult than anticipated to recruit faculty for the project were family pressures/responsibilities and fear. Participating in the Project meant being separated from family and friends for a month to a year or more. To make matters even worse, many of the courses taught by part-time faculty were scheduled from the middle of December to the middle of January. Teaching then meant being away from ones family during the Christmas and New Years holidays. The spouses of some potential faculty objected strongly to such a separation, particularly during the Holidays. In some cases, a family compromise was reached such that a spouse and/or children accompanied a faculty person to Gaza for the holiday teaching period .

There are several reasons why a faculty member could have declined to participate because of fear. When the project began, Gaza was under military occupation and the Intifada was still ongoing. There were frequent reports on CNN and other news services about fighting in Gaza between Israelis and Palestinians. These same news reports depicted Gaza and the refugee camps as being poverty-stricken war zones that were anything but a nice place to visit. Furthermore, the U.S. State Department had issued a warning about the safety of visiting the Gaza Strip. To make matters worse, the common U.S.-held stereotype of Palestinians was that of masked terrorists throwing rocks at Israelis on those days that they weren't bombing sites in Israel. Such preconceptions undoubtedly made potential faculty from the U.S. reluctant to participate in the Project. Incidentally, while many of the U.S. faculty and staff who participated in the Project acknowledged having some initial concerns about their safety, almost all of them reported that these concerns became insignificant shortly after arriving in Gaza. And after completing their time in Gaza, most of the Project's faculty reported that they would be willing to return.

When the Project was planned, the faculty for the speech-language pathology, audiology, and deaf education courses were to be primarily from Lamar University. While RM was fairly successful in recruiting Lamar University faculty for the audiology and deaf education courses, this was not the case for the speech-language pathology instructors. RM was forced to advertise nationally in a publication of the American Speech-Language-Hearing Association in 1993 for persons to teach these courses as adjunct Lamar University professors. FHS saw the advertisement a few months after participating in the First International Conference on Disability and Rehabilitation conducted by the Disabled Children Association in Riyadh, Kingdom of Saudi Arabia. This first experience in the Arab World had been such a positive one that, in spite of his being Jewish, he agreed to go to Gaza and teach three of the speech-language pathology courses.

Dr. Francis Lazarus was successful in recruiting faculty for the liberal arts core from persons associated with Marquette University. It was difficult for him to do so (for the reasons indicated elsewhere in this section) and both his dedication to the Project and his position as Vice President for Academic Affairs undoubtedly helped. Perhaps the most compelling evidence of his dedication to the Project was the fact that, in the summer of 1996, he accepted an administrative post at another university but then delayed his official departure from Marquette until he could participate in the graduation ceremony in Gaza and personally award diplomas to the Project graduates.

A few persons from countries other than the United States participated in the training program. A Jordanian woman taught Arabic sign language, a U.S.-trained professor from a Palestinian University in Gaza taught experimental phonetics, a U.S. trained Jordanian audiologist served as a consultant, and a Canadian served as a short-time audiologist.

ARRANGING "ROOM AND BOARD" FOR SHORT-TERM FACULTY

The SCHGS both owned and leased apartments and flats that had been used by the short-term faculty of its previous training programs. It also had a staffed central kitchen that had prepared meals for them. Both were used for this project.

Two meals a day usually were delivered to the apartments or flats of short-term faculty (the first around 7:00 a.m. and the other around 2:30 p.m). Each apartment and flat had a well-stocked refrigerator, a stove and/or microwave oven, and an adequate supply of bottled water. Both "American" and "Middle Eastern" food was available for breakfast. Faculty would occasionally go in small groups to one of the local restaurants for an evening meal.

The faculty would sometimes have their second meal together in a dining room at the SCHGS headquarters with Dr. Ghazaleh and his family. This happened most often when there were persons from Israel or the United States visiting the facility.

Each short-term faculty member was given a computer and printer to use at his or her apartment or flat. Both PCs with the Windows operating system and Apple Macintosh computers were available. The computers were set-up and maintained by an experienced technician who was employed by the Society.

MEETING FACULTY SECURITY NEEDS

The SCHGS took measures to ensure the safety of program faculty, particularly short-term ones. The Society had a fleet of vans, with professional drivers, that it used for transporting children to its various schools and other facilities. These vans were also used to transport faculty between their apartments or flats and the classroom building as well as to any other places to which they had to go in Gaza or Israel. Most of the faculty, at least a few times, did travel around Gaza by local taxi and/or walking and felt reasonably safe doing so.

RECRUITING NON-ACADEMIC SUPPORT STAFF

Most of the support staff (e.g., bus/van drivers, cleaning staff, technicians) were already in the employ of the SCHGS. Consequently, few had to be hired for the Project.

RECRUITING STUDENTS

In the Summer of 1992 the SCHGS placed an advertisement in local newspapers to recruit young men and women to be students in this Project. It described the program and indicated that persons selected to participate would have to be high school graduates, have good people skills, and be able to understand, speak, read, and write English well. At least 200 persons responded. We were unable to document the exact number, but it could have been as many as 400.

To save time, an initial screening of applicants to the Project was conducted by the SCHGS without the direct involvement of RM or others directly involved with the training program. Screening began in Gaza prior to the arrival of RM and the Project faculty. Persons who responded to the advertisement were given an application to complete in English. The application both asked for information about them and served as a screening device for their ability to read and write in English.

The applicants who appeared to be qualified to participate in the program (at least 120) were scheduled for an interview. The interviews were conducted individually in English by several persons associated with the SCHGS and by an American teacher of English as a second language. These interviews provided additional information about the applicants and (perhaps more importantly) their ability to both understand and speak English. The applicants were also administered a written English test.

About 80 of those interviewed were tentatively accepted for the program. At the onset, they were required to sign a document in which they acknowledged understanding and/or agreeing to the following:

- They will be attending classes for about three years
- All instruction will be in English

- They will not be allowed to smoke
- Low grades will not be acceptable in any course
- Failing even one course will result in expulsion from the program
- They will be required to work for the SCHGS for three years after they graduate

In November, 1992 they began an intensive three month English course that was taught by a teacher of English as a second language and by one of Dr. Ghazaleh's sons, who spoke English fluently. At the first session, Dr. Ghazaleh stated that he wanted to reduce the number of students in the program to 50 or fewer and their performance in this first course would be one of the ways he would do it. An examination was given to the students at the end of the course and, as a result of their performance on it, observations of their people skills, and other aspects of their behavior, the number of students in the program was reduced to 33 (25 men and 8 women).

COPING WITH STUDENT ENGLISH LANGUAGE DEFICIENCIES

Even after screening the students from several hundred to 33, many still did not have sufficient English to succeed in the Project unless they received help. Consequently, we decided to provide them with tutoring in English daily throughout the program. Two teachers of English as a second language were employed for this purpose.

Our decision to assist our students in developing their proficiency with English beyond the minimum required for our program has benefited them in a number of ways. It has, for example, enabled several of them to receive Fulbright and other scholarships for graduate study in England and in the United States.

COPING WITH THE NEED FOR MALE AND FEMALE STUDENTS TO ATTEND CLASSES TOGETHER

When the program began, it had been traditional in Gaza (and still is in most Arab countries) for male and female students to not attend class together. It would not have been practical for us to train the men and women separately. Consequently, for the first time in the Gaza Strip (or so we were told), men and women attended classes together. One result of our having them do this was at least half of the women falling in love with and marrying classmates, rather than having a traditional arranged marriage.

There was considerable social and even political pressure mitigating against our plans to teach young men and women in a coeducational program. In response to this pressure, the Project employed a mature woman referred to, only half in jest, as the "morals policeman." Though unspoken, it was understood that her job was to make sure that nothing culturally unacceptable occurred between the men and women students. Given the number of romances that occurred during the course of the Project, she wasn't all that effective.

COPING WITH DIFFERENCES (PERHAPS "CULTURAL") IN CLASSROOM BEHAVIOR

The similarities in classroom behavior of our students in Gaza to those in the States far outweighed the differences. There was, however, one significant difference. Our students in Gaza appeared to be more highly motivated than those in the States to help each other survive academically. While this attitude was commendable, it did cause problems during examinations at the beginning of the program. Stronger students quite openly attempted to help weaker ones. We indicated to the students that doing this was forbidden at American universities, and we separated them sufficiently during subsequent examinations to make doing it almost impossible. This ceased being a significant problem after the first course.

Chapter 3
The Students

The 33 Palestinian students in the program—25 men and 8 women—and their families resided in the Gaza Strip, almost all in refugee camps. Thirty-one were Moslems and two were Christians. Almost all were in their late teens or early 20s.

The information in the preceding paragraph only superficially answers the question, "Who were our students?" In order to be able to put at least a little "flesh on the bones" of whom they were, we did two things. First, we asked several of our graduates in November 2000 to respond by e-mail to the following question: "Who were you when the Program began and who are you now?" We've reproduced their responses (lightly edited) in the next section. And, second, we asked several of the faculty to answer the following question: "Who were your Palestinian students?" Some comments from their responses are also reproduced (lightly edited) here.

WHO WERE YOU WHEN THE PROGRAM BEGAN AND WHO ARE YOU NOW?

Akram E.

At the beginning of the program (and before it began) I lived in the AL Burij Refugee Camp in the Gaza Strip. I lived there with my parents, four brothers, and one sister. I am the second oldest of my brothers. During the Intifada, the educational system in the Gaza Strip was severely affected. In the 11th grade, I scored second highest in the whole school. It was really great that my efforts paid off. The exams were corrected by our teachers. The test scores were a valid estimate of my ability. However, in the 12th grade, our high school exams (Tawjehi) were corrected by the Egyptian Educational Ministry. There were some problems with exams during the Intifada. Complete schools were failed by the Egyptian Educational Ministry due to cheating. It was my fate to get 50% on the final high school exams. It was not a valid indicator of my ability. I decided to leave school because I would not be accepted by the local universities in a major that I like. My parents are really great. They inserted the following in our blood as children: EDUCATION IS THE WEAPON THAT YOU SHOULD HAVE FOR LIFE. It is a sentence that I will never forget .

I decided to work in Israel as a construction worker just to bury the frustration and depression that I had from the 50% result! My parents tried to force me to retake the high school exams. I would not listen. They knew that I studied well and trusted my ability.

I worked for approximately a year in Israel. I used to get to work at 3:00 in the morning and get back around 7:00 in the evening. It was a period that I hated. I VALUED EDUCATION HIGHLY. I decided to re-take the high school exams. Then I heard about the Program and that Dr. Abu Ghazaleh, the Director, was aware of what had occurred in Gaza education—i.e., that the marks students received during the Intifada were not necessarily a valid indicator of their abilities (something the local universities did not acknowledge at that time).

I applied and was accepted for the Program. It was the greatest day for me. I was back were I belonged. I did really well and received an *A* as a grade in all of the courses in my major. I scored at the top rank of the program, thanks to God.

Immediately after graduation, I was employed by the Society for the Care of the Handicapped in the Gaza Strip. It was great. I wanted to help my people. Audiology is something that I loved. I worked there for two years to gain experience. Then I worked at the Atfaluna Society for Deaf Children for two years.

Since graduating, I had been looking for a scholarship that would enable me to continue my education. It did not work out for one reason or another. I decided to get married in 1999. After I got married, I continued trying to get a scholarship to continue my education and eventually was successful in doing so. Let me tell you the truth. It came after I HAD GIVEN UP. My wife got pregnant and I had a son. I had to leave them to go to England to begin graduate study only 28 days after my son's birth in order to keep the scholarship. Deciding whether to do this was the toughest decision I ever had to make.

What have I accomplished professionally thus far? I established a screening program for preschool children at Atfaluna Society for Deaf Children. I supervised the establishment of at least one audiology clinic. I participated in several professional workshops in Gaza and Jerusalem. I served as a volunteer consultant for the Ministry of Health of the Palestinian Authority on hearing aids. I also served as a volunteer consultant for school primary health care with regard to hearing loss. I am currently working towards my masters in audiology in England and I hope that I'll be able help my people further when I go back.

Ramadan H.

I had been living in a refugee camp that is called Al Burij in the middle of the Gaza Strip. I had lots of dreams that had been limited by the occupation and by a very bad experience in my family with education. One of my brothers had failed his university study in India. I dreamed of being a neurosurgeon, however, I kept it as a dream. When I heard about the Program, I felt that it had the potential to make my dream of getting a university degree a reality. I registered for the program and loved it more and more with the passage of time.

Since graduating, I feel the proudness of my family in their eyes and I feel that I am a productive member of the society. Now I have stepped one step forward and I still have a dream to further my education.

By the way, I got married 4 months ago. My wife is beside me while I'm writing this e-mail. She is telling you that she is proud of me and my education.

Kamel A.

When I started the Program in Gaza/Palestine, I was a newly graduated student from high school. It was during the first Intifada, so our economic situation was very bad. My father was the only source of income for the family. He was working in Israel as a worker and there were six in the family. So it was very hard for him to pay the university costs. But my father insisted on his dream coming true to give me a chance to continue my education.

When I graduated in 1996, I could not find a good job to reduce the heavy load from my father shoulder because of the bad economic situation in the region. So I took a job at a tourism agency. I worked there for a year. Then I worked at a gas station for a week. Then I found a better job at a car dealership in Gaza. And finally, I found the good job that I have now. I work for the Orthodox Church as a public relations officer. I am also a volunteer for the Palestinian Speech and Hearing Association (PASHA), which is located in the Gaza Strip. Now that I have two jobs, one at the morning and the other on he afternoon, I'm a different man. And I'm happy that my father now works in Gaza rather than in Israel (in YMCA-Gaza), and he is happy that his dream to give me the opportunity to go to college came true.

Rae'da W.

I had finished high school and wanted to go to college. I heard about the program and it appealed to me. I also heard that all of the teaching would be in English. It was very difficult at the beginning because my English was limited. I tried hard to learn more English vocabulary at home. I wrote English words in a booklet and studied them. And I tried to learn English from the TV. My family encouraged me, especially my father. My father knew English well. He works in health research now. I improved my ability to speak and understand English, in part, by talking a lot with my professors.

I lived in a refugee camp, which is far from Gaza City (Nuseirat Camp). I had suffered a lot during the Intifada, but did my best to continue my studying. It was very difficult. I came to class even when there were strikes and the road was closed. [Not observing a strike called by Hamas was very dangerous and could result in injury or death. FHS] I had to study a lot. I spent most of the night studying because I spent so much time getting to and from class. I was away from home from 6:30 in the morning to 7:30 in the evening. I struggled a lot and my family did also. They did their best to help me and provide me with money. My education cost a lot more than my brothers and sisters. I had six sisters and four brothers and most of them were going to school at that time. Nobody in my family worked except my father. My family went without many things in order to be able to pay for our education.

Now, I am working as a speech-language pathologist in Gaza. The salaries in Gaza are low but working is better than staying at home. My family's situation is somewhat better now than in the past.

Nedal S.

On July 7, 1972, I was born in the Burij Refugee Camp at the middle of Gaza Strip. My mother and father were divorced. When I was four years old and my mother remarried, I moved to the Jabalia Refugee Camp, the most populous and the poorest of the camps in the Gaza Strip, to live with my grandparents (my father's parents), who raised me. My father married another woman and moved to Morocco.

I grew up under horrible circumstances. I was denied parental love and suffered, as one of the Palestinian people, the longest colonial occupation during the 20th century. As a child, I had emotional problems because of my parent's divorce as well as the economic, educational political and social situations that we all experienced. I went to an UNRWA elementary and junior high school. I'm proud of having done well in school despite all of my bad life circumstances.

In my first year at the high school, in 1987, the Palestinian Intifada erupted. Many of the martyrs during this Intifada (Dec. 9, 1987-Sep. 13, 1993) were of my fellow students and friends. Consequently, most of my generation underwent psychological stress and may still suffer the negative effects of the Intifada due to fear, imprisonment, beating, chasing, shooting, death etc. For me, I relentlessly tried to complete my studies in order to achieve my objectives and my dreams. I succeeded in finishing high school. But I felt confined by my fears and anxiety because of not being able to go to a college or a university that I liked as a result of my complicated social and family situations. Therefore, I lived the worst moments in my life.

When I learned about the Lamar Program that was to be inaugurated in Gaza City in cooperation with the Society for Handicapped (the Sun Center) in November 1992, I immediately headed there and briefed the administration about my difficult situation. They agreed to enroll me on the condition that I paid part of the tuition as soon as I could and promised to help me too. Indeed, being in the Program was one of the greatest and most interesting experiences in my life. I gained knowledge. I made friends. My personality was shaped. And I met a number of great and nice U.S. teachers (e.g., Dr. Robert Moulton, Dr. Smith, Mr. Sam Randazo, Dr. Frank Silverman, Miss Kathy Chinn and others.)

Now, I'm employed by the Fateh Foreign Relations Department, one of the Fateh institutions. (Fateh is the Arabic acronym that stands for Palestine National Liberation Movement, which is the main Palestinian political organization.) I have gotten married and God blessed me with a female child. Her name is Rana (1.5 yr.). Regarding my parents, each of them live their own life with their own family. I have no warm relations with my father, who lives in Gaza. On the other hand, I frequently visit my mother.

Finally, I'd like to thank Dr. F. Silverman particularly, and Marquette University generally, for the great efforts they made in conjunction with Lamar University to make it possible for my colleagues and I to get a university degree (B.S.). It has helped us to start and shape our future and what we learned has encouraged us to work for the best of our society.

Nasser Y.

When I was enrolled at the program, I was living with my family in a refugee camp (Beach Camp) near Gaza City and studying at the Islamic University, where you have your brain washed every day for five years. You only studied Islamic regulation. I hated it, but it was the only option for me. There was no other university in Gaza at that time. My dad did not like the idea of my going to the University. He wanted me to be a tailor. Because of the Intifada, the University was closed down, and economically, I could not afford to go to any other institution. Believe me, by that time I lost my hope of being able to get a university degree. Then, the Lord brought the Program to Gaza. [Nasser eventually left Gaza to study in England. He completed a master's degree there and was working on a second graduate degree when he died. See the addendum at the end of this chapter for a description of Nasser's life growing up in a refugee camp in Gaza.]

Mona A.

I was born in Gaza in September 1973 in a family of nine brothers and two sisters. I lived with my parents and youngest brother in Gaza City, very close to the Beach Camp for refugees. Most of my older brothers and my eldest sister had to work in the Gulf countries due to the shortage of employment opportunities in my country. I finished high school in 1991. I wanted to go to a university to continue my education, but I wasn't sure what I wanted to do. During that time, we were under great pressure from the Israeli occupation, Intifada, and limited access to universities. We couldn't study anything about our history, and the universities we had in Gaza weren't the greatest. Furthermore, it would have been difficult for me to go to a West Bank university because it was necessary to obtain some kind of permission from the military authority of the occupation. For these reasons, I had to stay in Gaza and find an educational opportunity there. My real chance came with the Lamar and Marquette program in communication disorder. This program was very beneficial and of great value to all of the students. It gave me new friends, new traditions, new knowledge and experience, and a huge opportunity to contact and help my community. During my undergraduate study, I developed skills in speech therapy, deaf education, aural rehabilitation, working with individuals with behavior problems, parent education and support, education of multidisabled persons, etc. This program made me a better person. It was great to have this program in our community where the position of disabled persons is considerably behind that in the industrialized countries.

One month after graduation I got married and moved to France, where my husband was finishing his PhD in tuberculosis research. In May 1997, we moved to Canada where he got a position at the University of Victoria. As soon as we arrived, I decided to pursue graduate study. At that time, I was interested in a masters degree in deaf education. However, I found that only five universities in Canada offered a masters degree in deaf education and the nearest one to me was the University of British Columbia in Vancouver. It would have been necessary for me to take the ferry between Victoria and Vancouver. This wasn't practical, especially because I had a baby. (I now have two children—Linda 3 years and Feras 10 months.) Therefore, I applied for admission to the masters program in special education at the University of Victoria.

Special education was the second field of interest for me. I was accepted provisionally into the special education program at the University of Victoria. They told me to take three courses to demonstrate my ability to do graduate work. I took the courses and got very good grades. However, at that time there was a funding problem in the lab where my husband worked. He had to look for another lab. He applied everywhere in Canada and got a good position in the Federal lab in Manitoba, where we live now. I didn't apply to the University of Manitoba because we found the city too cold, and I am not sure for how long we will be staying. My husband is thinking of moving to the USA because it's a better place for doing his kind of research. Now I am taking my fifth course in American sign language (ASL) and am still hoping to be able to get a masters degree. I have been contributing to the community where we live by volunteering at several large centers where I work with mentally challenged and hearing impaired children.

Mohammed, A.

I'm from a refugee camp. My family emigrated in 1948 from Ashdod, which is in the occupied territories, to Gaza to live in Beach Camp. My father works as a driver for the World Council of Churches. My family consist of 13 (eight sisters and two brother, me, and my mom and dad). When I entered the program, my father was the family's only source of income because my two brother were imprisoned in Israel (one of them had a life sentence). I spent the two years of my life after finishing the high school not studying at any university and because I wasn't interested in attending either of the two universities in Gaza and my father didn't have money to pay for me to study abroad.

Now I work for the UNDP, the United Nation Development Program. I get a good salary in comparison to the average income in Gaza. I'm married and have a son. My wife is Samar El R., one of the students from the Program. She works for the UN. We have an apartment that is fully furnished, and a car in moderately good condition. My parents' situation is also getting better. They built a new house and I give my father some money every month to help them. I'm now well known among the non-governmental organizations in Gaza. It's become somewhat easier for me to find job opportunities. I have mostly worked on short-term projects since I graduated—every year or two I have changed jobs. Since graduating, I have acquired many new skills, had many new experiences, taken many courses, and attended many national and international conferences.

Ashraf Y.

In 1990 after finishing high school I went to Amman, Jordan to pursue my education. But I was not able to complete it because of financial problems and returned to Gaza. After doing so, I worked on construction in Israel for a living. I wanted to continue my education, but the local colleges did not offer training that met my needs. When I heard about this program from my brother, who was working at The Sun Day Care Center, I rushed down and enrolled.

It was very challenging and encouraging at the same time. It raised my self-esteem. It helped me to become more open-minded and a more logical thinker. It was a unique program that offered an education with such high standards that it caused most students in the local universities to envy us.

Three months after graduation, I took a position as a supervisor in the Right To Live Society which serves Down's Syndrome children in Gaza. I then worked at another institution as a supervisor. In both places, I was asked to give presentations to the staff about speech problems.

Marquette University provided a high level of education that helped me a great deal. It not only helped me in the field of speech therapy, it helped me with English as well. I ended up with a knowledge of English sufficient to work as a professional translator. I translated research on Palestinian ex-prisoners' experiences and the effect of the political situation in Gaza on school-age children living there for the Gaza Community Mental Health Program.. I also helped to facilitate the training of a group of Palestinian women on how to synthesize a questionnaire, for a study of women living in Gaza. The training was performed by a Professor from Helsinki University in Finland who did not speak Arabic and the trainees did not speak English.

Samar R.

My family and I are refugees. I have four brothers and five sisters. We emigrated from a village called Masmia in 1948. My family lived in Jabalia refugee camp for a couple of years and then moved to Gaza City down town and then to Saudia Arabia, where I was born. We lived in Saudia Arabia until the late 80's. My father worked there as a teacher and in other businesses. My family saved some money and come back to Gaza and opened a very small business. So our financial situation during the time before I entered the university was fairly good in comparison with most of the People in Palestine. We lived in a modern area of Gaza City. When I finished high school, I refused to study at any of the universities that existed in Gaza at the time. Unfortunately, my father was not able to pay for my study abroad at that time because two of my brothers were in college. I was out of high school for two years before I was accepted for the Program. I learned a lot during my study in addition to information about the field. And moreover, I met my husband while in the Program. He was also a student in it. And we married before graduating.

Now I work for UNRWA as a Credit Extension Assistant. And soon I will be an officer. I'm married and happy with my husband Mohammed and my son. We have an apartment with good furniture and a car. I feel that it was a wonderful opportunity for me to get my education in this Program. And I feel that it raised my life up.

WHO WERE YOUR PALESTINIAN STUDENTS?

The comments reproduced here were abstracted from e-mail and other documents that we requested and received from participating faculty to help "flesh out" who our students were.

- I had worked with Israeli students before, in this country,...and I liked them very much because they were eager, hardworking, bright, and receptive to instruction. I found the Palestinians the same, maybe the most eager students I have ever worked with.
- They were one level higher than almost every student I've had.
- One often feels...at an American University that one is a kind of add-on to a certification process, not really an educator. Or that one represents a requirement that students must somehow survive. I found among the Palestinian students a genuine interest in finding out what liberal arts education really is.
- The students are making progress and follow my lectures with much more interest than American students. They are always stopping me and asking for clarification and when I make good points, I have their rapt attention.
- The next day's topic was literature. I asked people to bring stories or poems that they liked, and I brought some as well. Mine were personal, but theirs were more so. It turned out that one of our thirty-three is well known in Gaza—along with literally dozens of others—as a poet worth listening to. Some days later, when he had written a new poem, almost the entire group gathered around him during their break to hear him present it. No matter how rudimentary their training they told me, in their early years all had memorized large portions of the Koran, and not surprisingly they took away his new poem in their heads. This is apparently standard—any of them could have given me poems by the score, translating as they went through them. Now who was teaching literature to whom? And in whose culture is poetry more alive?
- Teaching is vastly different, exhausting and delightful. These are really fine students. They have maintained their joy of life amid terrible adversity....They are totally engaged in the process of learning.
- Almost all of the students evinced a great deal of interest in Palestinian politics. Many of the men had participated in the Intifada. In fact, we

were told that 24 of the 25 had been jailed by the Israelis (in at least one case for as long as two years) for activities during it. The student who wasn't said to have been jailed by them, incidentally, received a master's degree in 1999 from the Department of Politics at York University in England. Because of our students' strong interest in politics and their leadership abilities, I believe that at least a few of them are likely to assume major leadership roles in a future Palestinian state or whatever Palestinian political entity eventually develops.

ADDENDUM

One of the students in the Program, Nasser Y., died in England in 1999 after completing one masters degree (in political science) and while working on another. Nasser's childhood was probably typical, in at least some ways, of that of our other students who grew up in a refugee camp. In July, 1998, he e-mailed one of us (FHS) a portion of a story about his childhood entitled *A Bed of Roses (So you think you've got it rough?)* that had been written by a Canadian journalist to whom Nasser had given Arabic lessons. Unfortunately, Nasser didn't include the name of the journalist or the newspaper for whom the journalist worked. Consequently, it wasn't possible to seek permission from the copyright holder to reproduce portions of the article here. Since these excerpts provide some insight into what life was like in a refugee camp in Gaza when our students were children and consequently, into who our students were, we hope that the author and publisher will consider our inclusion of material from this article to be both for the public good and consistent with the doctrine of "fair use."

****

Nasser Y. is a 30 year old Palestinian who has lived in Beach Camp in the Gaza Strip for almost all of his life. I got to know him as my Arabic instructor, but he worked full time as a support staff person for a UN agency in Gaza City. He has trained and worked as a speech-language therapist, and had a variety of jobs before this—from taxi driver to interpreter for foreign language press during the Intifada. Now Nasser is trying to get a scholarship to study abroad to pursue his interest in international relations as it relates to the Palestinian situation today.

The real story, however, is how Nasser got to where he is today. And the road he has traveled to reach his present location is a particularly rocky one, at least compared to the four lane superhighways that most Canadians cruise along.

Nasser's history has been shaped by several factors that are not part of the experience, or even present in the consciousness, of 95 percent of native-born Canadians.

These include, first of all, the family social structure, which is dominated by the father. The relationship between the father and the rest of the family in traditional Gaza households is based very much on the indisputable fact that the father and husband is in charge. Whatever he says goes, no questions asked or considered. This clear dominance can be an advantage or disadvantage, depending on where you sit in the pecking order and the way in which the head of the household wields his authority. The men can't be blamed totally for the very autocratic way in which they act. They are playing out a role that is expected of them by their society—or at least the other men in it.

A second major influence on everyone's life in the Gaza Strip has been the Israeli presence—from the mass exodus of refugees from Israel in 1949, to the Israeli occupation of Gaza in 1967, to the Intifada from 1986-93, to the stalled peace talks today. Every Palestinian has lived and breathed and suffered at the hands of the state of Israel for most of their lives.

Finally, and perhaps most significantly for Nasser, is his disability. A common theme throughout his life has been trying, and succeeding, to prove to others that he can accomplish as much and do better a job than his able-bodied colleagues. His story is evidence of how well he has met his challenge.

For Nasser, the story starts with his family's flight from a small town between Yaffa and Ashkelon in 1948 to the Gaza Strip, following the defeat of the neighboring Arab countries by the newly founded state of Israel. In their original community, Nasser's grandfather had been the largest landowner and obviously well off. Fleeing from their home to Gaza landed them at the other end of the wealth spectrum—impoverished with no belongings and little money. Nasser's father made some money at first selling gas for stoves and lamps and then worked for a long period as a plasterer. However, a tumor in his lower back 18 years ago forced him out of work for an extended period. He eventually went back to work on light construction in Israel, but found that is physical condition was not good enough to continue strenuous labor. So he stopped, and since that time has relied on the income provided by the rest of his family.

During this period, his wife bore 15 children—eight sisters and seven brothers—now aged from 18 to 38. His mother started a small business sewing clothes for neighborhood women. Overall the history of her experience in raising her family, running a small business and living with the typical demands of a Gazan husband and large family is probably worth a separate account, but I am only aware of it from what I have learned about Nasser's own history.

My introduction to Nasser's story began one day when he mentioned to me, with some mirth, that a child in his neighborhood had been so bold as to challenge his father's treatment of his family, especially Nasser's younger brother. The child, who I later learned was 18, had told Nasser's father openly how badly he was mistreating his son, apparently by beating him with little or no reason. He dared Nasser's father to beat him for his temerity but the father was too stupefied by such blatantly unacceptable behavior to respond. A few questions on my part to try to understand better what was going on presented me with a better understanding of Nasser's overall life experience, including life with an omnipotent father....I didn't learn much about how Nasser's father had treated his brother but I got to know quite a bit about how Nasser fared under his father's not so benevolent guardianship and in the general environment of life in Gaza under Israeli occupation.

Nasser's life has not been a bed of roses by Canadian standards and from early childhood it was much more thorns than blossoms. First of all, Nasser contracted polio when he was two years old....The pretty minimal health care available in the refugee camps in the Gaza Strip during the 1960's did not cover widespread vaccination campaigns that by then were the norm in the developed world. The bottom line for Nasser was that he was left with severely deformed legs.

He then spent four years in a rehabilitation center in Jerusalem where he underwent operations to correct as much as possible the mis-alignment of his legs and feet due to polio. He remembers being anaesthetized before the operation by having a cloth placed over his face and chloroform being poured onto directly over his nose. When he awoke, he would have his leg in a cast. He also remembered the terror he felt when he was first approached by a Nurse with a small electric saw to remove the cast, and he thought that it was to remove his leg—cast and all. After four years it was over though, and Nasser returned home to live with his family in Gaza.

This physical challenge was only the start for Nasser. Living in Beach Camp in general...proved just as testing as the disability brought on by polio.

Beach Camp is a small area—less than a square kilometer—but with more than 60,000 residents now. As with most refugee families, getting by in the camp was a daily challenge that required everyone to contribute.

Nasser's disability didn't stop him from having to perform a variety of chores for his family and doing his bit to assist. He described how one of his first chores was cleaning the soot from the glass of the kerosene lamps in his home every morning. He also spent days unraveling scrap cloth. The strands would then be used to stuff home-made mattresses and pillows. There certainly wasn't money for buying such items.

More demanding was tending to the chicks, ducks, and pigeons that his father raised. His father wanted the chicks to get plenty of sun and the only place to find this was in the narrow street between the houses. So it was Nasser's job to tend the flock while they sunned themselves. The problem was that chicks, often 100 in number, were rather prone to wondering. Keeping them in one spot would have been a challenge for anyone. It was more difficult for Nasser as he did not yet have crutches but got around by using a stool as a substitute for crutches. He would keep the stool in front of him and push it forward to provide support as he moved about as best he could. But chasing chickens in this fashion was impossible. Nasser was fairly creative, though, and he fashioned a makeshift lasso from a piece of rope and a stone. As he sat on the stool he would whip the lasso out at any chicks that tried to stray off. This was somewhat effective but Nasser recalls that he spent a lot of time sitting on the stool and crying because of the impossible task he had and how difficult life would be if his father felt that any chicks were missing.

When he was seven years old, he and his sister would walk, he on crutches, for several kilometers along the road early on Friday mornings, their day off school. The would collect up scraps of paper and other materials for fuel in the clay oven his mother used to bake bread.

They soon graduated to more lucrative work. At 4:00 am on Friday mornings they would travel the same distance to the dock in front of Gaza City. There they would help the fishermen unload their catch in the morning. Nasser recalled how heavy the crates of fish were and what hard work it was. For their efforts they would get a handful of fish. It was a bit of a free for all with helpers moving quickly from one boat to the next to unload their catch. Because of his small size and his crutches, Nasser sometimes got extra handfuls from the fishermen on other boats that he hadn't exactly helped unload. Then they would try to beg a ride back to Beach Camp on a donkey cart. Otherwise they had to drag their sack of fish home to add to the family larder.

Making ends meet in Nasser's home during this period involved quite a bit of ingenuity. His mother used to have the children play a game to compensate for the lack of food in the house. She would ask them to see how long they could make a single olive last at meal time—the meal consisting of a single olive and bread. The winner would get an extra piece of bread. Nasser recalls licking the olive and smelling it and trying to stretch out its life to win the game. What this nutritional game did for their mental health is unknown, but it certainly wouldn't help in building strong bodies and agile minds. This main meal was supplemented by the lunches Nasser would take to school every day—bread with hot peppers; this certainly would put spice into the school day but not much else.

During this period Nasser was attending school. He remembered when he was nine years old finishing first in his class. However, he dreaded his accomplishment. It was the custom at the school that the student who finished first in class would have to treat the other students to chocolates. Nasser knew that his father wouldn't pay for the chocolates and he had no money of his own. After he was formally recognized as the top student in his class, his classmates harassed him for several days for their chocolates. He spent three days crying at home and eventually went to his mother to beg her for money for chocolates. She got it for him by borrowing money from a neighbor—six shekels, $2.50 today and probably a lot of money 20 years ago, especially in a refugee camp. Nasser took the chocolates to school but he didn't get full marks for his efforts—the chocolates weren't the kind that they wanted; he only had enough money to buy a cheaper brand. His teacher reinforced the students' feelings by telling Nasser that his family was very stingy—just the sort of positive feedback that is likely to encourage students to higher academic achievement.

Nasser did draw top marks from his classmates when it came to soccer. He was much sort after to play goalkeeper. He was quick and able to block shots with his crutches that would have been out of the reach of the kids who didn't have the advantage of his disability. He could also use the crutches to control the ball very well in goal mouth scrambles.

Nasser got his first taste of full-time employment when he was eleven. For three years he spent his summers working for a tailor. He had learned how to use a sewing machine from his mother. The owner of the shop he worked for was amazed by how quickly Nasser learned the business. Nasser didn't tell him how he had gained his skills—he wanted to impress the owner than he could do good work despite his disability. In return for his hard work the owner gave Nasser some money—an amount decided upon by the owner. It would have been inappropriate for Nasser to ask for any compensation. Nasser then handed the money over to his father, for which gesture he earned some measure of respect....

Nasser finished secondary school at 18 and that was the end of the line as far as Nasser's father was concerned. Now it was time to stop playing and to work in earnest. Nasser went to work as a tailor but he wanted to continue his education. He made an agreement with his boss to allow him to use a sewing machine at home. He spent his first year as the Islamic University in Gaza going to school in the morning and returning home by 1:00 p.m. Then he would work at the sewing machine for a full shift until 1:00 a.m. in the morning. His reward for this effort was his father's refusal to allow Nasser to continue this routine any longer after his first year of college. However, Nasser took the highly unusual and drastic action of leaving home. Tired of the physical and verbal abuse which he had suffered throughout his life, he moved out of his father's house and went to work in a restaurant in Israel. After one and a half years he returned to Gaza to continue his education. He still worked in the restaurant in Israel on weekends and did other jobs on the side....

Attending college without a home was not a picnic however. Nasser had brought a car in 1986 with money he made from serving as an interpreter for foreign journalists. He used the car as a taxi to earn enough income to cover his tuition and other expenses while at school....His home was his taxi. When he wasn't driving it to pick up fares, he parked it in a garage he had rented in Remal area in Gaza City and slept in it. Remal is a well-to-do neighborhood and was rarely bothered by the Israeli Defense Force during the Intifada. Here he would take out a blanket and drape it over himself to block out any light. Then he would use a flashlight to read his books and study for school. The taxi also served as his kitchen.

Chapter 4
Implementation

The program began at the end of 1992 and the students graduated with their bachelor's degrees in July of 1996. A number of tasks had to be performed prior to and/or during this period to implement the program. Several, including the securing of grant funding and the recruitment of students, have been dealt with previously. In this chapter we describe, somewhat candidly, a number of the other aspects of the implementation for our program. It is our hope that some of this information will be helpful to those who are planning similar programs in other fields and/or in other developing countries.

ACQUIRING AND EQUIPPING FACILITIES

One of the first tasks that had to be done was to acquire and equip the facilities needed to implement the Program. These included classrooms, practicum facilities, and a library. These facilities and how they were acquired and equipped are described here.

Classrooms

The classroom facility that was used for this program was on the first floor of a building that the Society for the Care of the Handicapped in the Gaza Strip (SCH) had leased and had remodeled and equipped for its previous rehabilitation personnel training programs, including one (for which it had partnered with the University of Calgary in Canada) that was being conducted when this program began. It contained two regular classrooms, one of which could accommodate at least 20 students and the other at least 35. It also contained a large room that served as a library and, when needed, a third classroom. Other facilities included a room containing PCs (with Windows Operating Systems) for student use, a large reception room, faculty offices, a faculty lounge, and a student lounge. There was also a courtyard where students "could let off steam" (e.g., by tossing a Frisbee) between classes. On the second floor was a medical facility.

The furnishings in the classrooms and the audio/visual equipment available for instructional purposes were comparable to those available to instructors on their home campuses. The latter included slide projectors, overhead projectors, videotape players with large monitors, audiotape recorders, computers, and sophisticated photocopy machines for duplicating handouts.

One rather unusual piece of equipment was a fairly powerful portable electric generator. The Gaza Strip (in whole or part) experienced frequent disruptions in electric service during the period that we were conducting our program. They were, in some cases, deliberate. For instance, the Israelis might turn off the power to an entire city block if one resident of the block refused to pay a utility bill. Then too, the Israelis might turn off the power in Gaza in response to a political protest, bombing, strike, etc.

Practicum Facilities

An important aspect of the training programs in speech-language pathology, audiology, and deaf education was supervised clinical and/or teaching experience. There were no facilities in the Gaza Strip for providing such experience when the program began. It was, therefore, necessary to construct (or remodel) and equip facilities for providing all three types of practicum experience. These facilities, of course, were also a community resource because they facilitated the delivery of diagnostic, therapeutic, and educational assistance to communicatively-impaired children and adults in the Gaza Strip.

Audiology. A floor was added to the Sun Day Care Center (the Society for the Care of the Handicapped in the Gaza Strip's main facility) to house the audiology clinic. It contained several high quality hearing testing suites as well as facilities for counseling patients and doing hearing rehabilitation, including dispensing hearing aids. All of the equipment utilized for audiometric testing and rehabilitation was state-of-the art.

The hearing testing suites were hand-made yet still met ANSI standards. By the time we got these built, however, we were wishing that we had purchased IAC booths in the United States and shipped them to Gaza. The local craftsmen who built them had never seen or experienced a sound-controlled environment.

Speech-Language Pathology and Deaf Education. Initially, Gazans needing audiology, speech-language pathology, and/or deaf education services came to the Sun Day Care Center where our faculty and our students provided services. Then, in 1994, a building was leased and remodeled to serve as a speech and language disorders and deaf education practicum facility. Though relatively small, it was comparable in quality to those utilized by most universities in the States for providing these types of practicum experience. It contained several large rooms that could be used for either group therapy or classes for deaf children. Several of the rooms had large one-way observation mirrors. The electronic equipment available for speech and language rehabilitation and teaching deaf children was comparable in quality to that utilized for practicums in these fields at most U.S. universities.

Because the Project was funded by a grant from the United States government, we were required to purchase equipment and supplies in the United States even though the same (or similar) equipment and supplies were often available in nearby Israel. We shipped it to Gaza or ask Project personnel traveling from the U.S. to Gaza to serve as "mules." Many times, short-term faculty would bring a few hundred pounds of texts and supplies with them as luggage.

Library Facilities

The classroom facility that was utilized for this program contained a one-room library that was reasonably well equipped (including tables at which students could sit and study). It did not, however, have an adequate collection of journals and books in speech-language pathology, audiology, or deaf education or in most of the liberal arts areas in which the students took courses. Consequently, instructors had to bring with them any books (other than textbooks) and articles that they needed to teach their courses.

As far as we knew, there was no adequate collection of journals and books in speech-language pathology, audiology, or deaf education anywhere in the Gaza

Strip. There were such collections at university libraries in Israel, but our students didn't have access to them.

ACQUIRING ARABIC THERAPY/TEACHING MATERIALS AND DIAGNOSTIC TESTS FOR PRACTICUMS

Acquiring such materials for speech-language pathology practicums was more of a problem than it was for deaf education and audiology ones. Some materials for teaching Arabic Sign Language had been developed in Jordan and elsewhere in the Arab world, including Palestine. [In an earlier United Nations-funded (UNDP) project, incidentally, RM participated in the development of what may well have been the first dictionary of the Arab Sign Language.] Our students were trained with teaching materials for both the Jordanian and Palestinian "dialects" of Arabic Sign Language.

The lack of Arabic materials for audiology practicums was not a severe problem. The only types of hearing tests that were impacted were those that used speech as stimuli—for example, ones for establishing the Speech Reception Threshold (SRT). Arabic "first approximations" of such stimuli were developed by faculty and students in the Project.

The lack of Arabic testing and therapy materials impacted significantly on our speech-language pathology practicums. While at least "first approximations" of some such materials had undoubtedly been developed by speech-language pathologists in Arabic-speaking countries, they had not, to the best of our knowledge, been published either in professional journals or by test/material publishers. Consequently, it was necessary for our students to create Arabic adaptations of some such tests and materials from English ones. Such adaptations included substituting culturally-appropriate for culturally-inappropriate test stimuli (e.g., drawings or photographs). These adaptations were, of course, only "first approximations" and, as such, needed to be refined and, if tests, standardized also.

PROCURING FACULTY

The long-term faculty consisted mostly of licensed (and/or certified) practitioners from the United States in audiology, deaf education, speech-language pathology, and teaching English as a second language. Most of the short-term faculty were associated with either Lamar University or Marquette University as a professor, an adjunct professor, a clinical supervisor, or a graduate student. A few of the short-term faculty taught at other institutions in the United States, Canada, the Gaza Strip, or Jordan. Incidentally, with the exception of the few faculty from the Middle East, none were able to speak Arabic fluently.

One of us (RM) had the primary responsibility for recruiting the faculty (both long-term and short-term) other than the ones from Marquette University who taught the liberal arts core courses. The latter were recruited by Dr. Francis Lazarus who, at the time, was Marquette's Vice President for Academic Affairs.

Most of the long- and the short-term faculty from the U.S. who taught professional courses were recruited by RM in one of two ways. They were either recruited from Lamar University faculty and graduate students or from responses to advertisements that RM had placed in professional journals.

Dr. Lazarus went "far beyond the call of duty" when recruiting faculty for teaching the 18 course liberal arts core. Because he believed strongly in the Program, recruiting faculty for it became a priority for him. The fact that he was Marquette's Vice President for Academic Affairs undoubtedly influenced the decision of some faculty to participate. As we've indicated previously, perhaps the most compelling evidence of his commitment to the program was his decision to delay his resignation from Marquette (to accept an upper administrative position at another university) until a few hours after the graduation ceremony in Gaza so that he would be able to officiate at it.

The relationship between each person who taught in the Program and the Society for the Care of the Handicapped (SCH) was formalized by a "Letter of Agreement." A typical one for a short-termer is reproduced in Appendix E.

MEETING THE PERSONAL NEEDS OF FACULTY

To attract and retain faculty, it was necessary to meet their personal as well as professional needs. Long-term faculty would be likely to resign if their personal needs weren't being met. And it would become increasingly difficult to recruit short-term faculty if word got out that this was the case. Some of the ways that these needs were met are described in this section.

"Room and Board"

Long-term faculty lived either in apartments that were owned or leased by the Society or in ones in Gaza City that were privately owned. They had to purchase and prepare their own food and be responsible for meeting their other personal needs. They would, of course, have also had to assume these responsibilities if they were working in the States. There were stores throughout Gaza City where food and other necessities could be purchased.

Short-term faculty were housed in apartments that were owned or leased by the Society. They were provided with two meals a day (one at about 7:00 a.m. and the other at about 2:30 p.m.). They were also provided with bottled water as well as soft drinks, instant coffee, tea, milk, fruit (including delicious tangerines), yogurt, eggs, cheese, pita bread, corn flakes, and other foods for snacks.

Security

Security was a serious concern, particularly at the beginning of the program (the Gaza Strip was still under Israeli occupation and the Intifada was ongoing). Automatic weapon fire was heard by participating faculty throughout the period that the Program was conducted. During much of it, there was an armed guard seated outside the main gate to the Sun Center, where most of the short-term faculty were housed. Furthermore, partially because of security concerns, short-term faculty were transported by van from their apartments to and from the classroom building, the Sun Center, and wherever else they had to go in Gaza for professional reasons.

The short-term faculty were not encouraged to travel around Gaza City on their own. However, many did so (including the authors). To the best of our knowledge, none had life-threatening experiences while doing so. However, a few of our female faculty did have unpleasant experiences when traveling around Gaza City on their own, without their hair being covered (a requirement of the traditional Moslem dress code for women).

Transportation

Round-trip business class tickets (on TWA) to Tel Aviv were provided for participating short-term faculty by the Society for the Care of the Handicapped in the Gaza Strip. The Society also provided airline tickets for long-term faculty. Arriving faculty were met at the airport by a representative of the Society who transported them by van to Gaza City. Departing faculty were transported by van to the Tel Aviv airport, usually at least five hours early. This was necessary because persons who had been in the Gaza Strip were often subjected to a lengthy security interrogation before being permitted to go to their departure gate.

As we've indicated previously, short-term faculty were transported by van wherever they had to go in the Gaza Strip for professional reasons. This type of transportation was also provided occasionally for sight-seeing in Gaza and Israel.

Teaching Preparation

Short-term faculty were provided with computers and printers for preparation of materials for teaching or whatever else they wanted to do with them. Some faculty, for example, used them for keeping diaries (see Appendix C), writing manuscripts, and/or meeting ongoing responsibilities on their home campuses. Recent models of both Macintosh computers and PCs with a Windows Operating System were available. A very knowledgeable computer technician was also available to solve any software or hardware problems.

Sophisticated photocopy machines for duplicating tests and handouts were available at both the classroom building and the Sun Center. A fax machine was also available at the Sun Center for securing information needed for teaching from the States.

Recreation

U.S.-style recreational opportunities in Gaza were limited. Short-term faculty were sent to Gaza at least two at a time so that they would have somebody to talk to. Married faculty were allowed to bring their spouses. Groups of faculty occasionally went to a local restaurant for an evening meal. All of the apartments had television sets, but the language in almost all of the programs was Arabic. The Project had a library of paperback novels, left behind by previous faculty persons and added to by each new or returning instructor. The director of the program occasionally invited short-term faculty to his home for a meal. Some opportunities for sight-seeing in Gaza and Israel were usually provided. The U.N. had a social club (the Beach Club) in Gaza with a bar and restaurant that some faculty went to. However, going there was discouraged because they discriminated against Palestinians. That is, Palestinians were not invited to join the Beach Club so, as a means of making a statement against this policy, some Project faculty refused to join the club or otherwise participate in its activities.

While official Project policy discouraged the faculty from socializing with the students (e.g., visiting the students' homes and meeting their families), many did so (including both authors). Palestinians tend to be very hospitable people and the students did what they could to make the stays of both the short- and long-termers as pleasant as possible. Many friendships were establish between Project students and faculty that have endured (mostly via e-mail) to the present.

PROCURING LOCAL SUPPORT STAFF

The various types of local support staff that were needed to implement our Program were already in place when it began because the University of Calgary's programs were still going on and ours utilized the same facilities (and, in a few cases, even the same faculty).

DEVELOPING ADEQUATE RECORD-KEEPING SYSTEMS

It was necessary for both the accounting and student record-keeping systems to be consistent with United States standards because the Project was being funded by the United States Government (USAID) and degrees were being awarded by an American university. Some comments relevant to their implementation are presented in this section.

Accounting

USAID had many rules regarding how grant funds could and could not be spent. It was necessary for the Society to significantly modify some of the budgets in the grant while it was ongoing for at least two reasons. First, funding for the Marquette University 18 semester hours of liberal arts courses was not part of the Project's initial budget. That is, there was no mention of or provision for Marquette's involvement in the 1992 budget, but Marquette was part of the 1994 budget. And second, in 1994 when the Israeli occupation of most of the Gaza Strip ended, the Palestinian Authority employed a police force to fill the vacuum left by the departed Israelis. Some of the funding for this new police force came from a USAID decision to reduce the Project budget and transfer the funds to the Palestinian Authority.

The manner in which the Society "creatively" reallocated funds to make it possible to fund the Marquette component of the Program and to complete the Project with less funding than was originally allocated brought it into conflict with auditors from USAID. The Society also appears to have had some conflict with USAID over what constitutes standard and/or ethical business practices.

What is generally regarded as being an unacceptable business practice in one culture may be generally regarded as being an acceptable one in another!

Student Records

Since the students were to receive regular Bachelor of Science degrees from the College of Communication at Marquette University, the academic records that were maintained on them were essentially the same as those maintained on other students who were working on this degree in the College of Communication at Marquette's main campus. The speech-language pathology, audiology, and deaf education courses that they took from regular and adjunct faculty from Lamar University were accepted as equivalent to ones required for the undergraduate major in the Department of Speech Pathology and Audiology at Marquette University. The semester credit hours associated with the professional courses taken by Project students exceeded Marquette's requirements for speech pathology and audiology majors.

DEVELOPING RULES REGARDING CLASS ATTENDANCE AND PERFORMANCE, CHEATING, AND OTHER ACADEMIC ISSUES

Rules regarding these were developed and strictly enforced.

ORIENTING FACULTY

Each faculty member received a "Welcome to Gaza Packet" handout before going there the first time (see Appendix D). We decided to include this handout as an appendix both because it provides some insight into the environment in which the faculty functioned and can serve as a model for such packets for future programs of this type.

Some faculty were also oriented informally before going there by ones who had been there previously. This was particularly true for liberal arts faculty from Marquette University.

SECURING "COMMUNITY" SUPPORT

Considerable attention was given to acquainting the leadership of the Palestinian Authority with the Program in order to secure its support. Dr. Hatem met a number of times with President Arafat and his Minister of Health to acquaint them with the Program and secure their help. President Arafat's wife and members of the Palestinian Authority toured the Program's clinics and other facilities. President Arafat met several times with Project faculty at his headquarters in Gaza and agreed to be the commencement speaker at the Project's graduation ceremony.

An attempt was also made to acquaint persons in the "rehabilitation community" in Israel with the Program and hopefully secure their support for it and its graduates. Some Israeli rehabilitation specialists toured the Program's clinics and other facilities. Information about the Program, particularly the deaf education aspect of it, was presented at conferences in Israel. An Israeli specialist in deaf education from Tel Aviv University was a guest lecturer for us in Gaza, an unheard of event! On one occasion, Project faculty met with more than a dozen Israeli communicative disorders specialists at a motel in Beersheba. The purpose of this meeting was to discuss problems associated with Israeli-Arab citizens who have communication disorders.* And a philanthropic organization in Israel was sufficiently impressed with the program to explore the possibility of replicating it in the West Bank.

Some attempt was also made to acquaint the rehabilitation community in Jordan with the Program. A U.S.-trained Jordanian audiologist lectured in the Program as did a Jordanian teacher of the deaf. And a meeting was arranged in Jordan between Program faculty and that of a Jordanian school for the deaf but the meeting had to be canceled because of travel restrictions.

SCHEDULING COURSES

The students took courses during the summer, as well as during the academic year. And they also took courses during the December-January semester break period. The primary reason why courses were scheduled during the summer and the semester break period was that these were the only times that many short-term faculty could come to Gaza to teach.

The students were required to attend class six days a week. And they were required to be "on campus" as many as ten hours a day. For the courses that all of the students took, they were divided into two groups—one consisted of 16 and the other of 17 students. Group assignment was not based on ability. The classes in each such course were taught twice the same day. When two courses, for example, were scheduled for a morning, while one instructor taught his or her course to

* Also, on this occasion, Project faculty met with a group of Bedouin-Israelis who had a much greater than normal rate of congenital deafness.

Group A the other taught his or hers to Group B. Then, after a short break the students switched classrooms and had a class in the other course. Classes usually lasted about two hours. It was decided to have two groups so that each student would have ample opportunity to ask questions and participate in class discussions. Many of the instructors commented that these students did considerably more of both than did those on their home campuses.

INCREASING ENGLISH LANGUAGE PROFICIENCY

The knowledge of English of many of our students, particularly at the beginning of the program, was barely adequate. To at least partially remedy this situation, we did the following throughout the program. First, we required students to take a class in English as a second language almost every day. We employed two full-time teachers of English as a second language at the beginning of the program and one at the end.** The students liked and respected both and this helped a lot.

Incidentally, the proficiency with English that many of the students gained from the program contributed significantly to their employment options following graduation. In fact, a few who were unable to find a job in Gaza as a speech-language pathologist, audiologist, or teacher of the deaf after graduation worked as translators.

COPING WITH CULTURAL DIFFERENCES IN CLASSROOM BEHAVIOR

The students' interaction in the classroom with both faculty and peers differed significantly from what is usual in the United States, particularly at the beginning of the Program. They talked with each other almost constantly during class and asked many more questions than faculty usually got when they taught the same course on their home campus (see Appendix C). And during examinations, the stronger ones sometimes tried to help the weaker ones pass.

While we recognized that some of the "undesirable" differences in classroom behavior could be cultural, we nevertheless felt it necessary to get them to conform as much as possible to expectations for students in the United States. This was done, in part, to enhance the comfort level of faculty. We were successful in controlling the students' attempts to help each other during examinations by

** We discovered that a good source for such teachers is Peace Corps veterans. We advertised in a Peace Corps journal and found a ready supply of TOESL wannabees.

indicating to them that doing so was unacceptable at American universities and by spreading them out and closely monitoring them whenever they took an examination. We were less successful in getting their behavior during lectures to conform to that of students in the States. However, a number of instructors did comment that, although the students' almost continuous questioning at times got on their nerves, their genuine enthusiasm for learning made them a delight to teach.

CREDENTIALING GRADUATES

The Program began as one in which the students were to be credentialed by a certificate from Lamar University. However, it ended up as one in which the credential they received was a Bachelor of Science degree from the College of Communication at Marquette University, the same degree that undergraduate majors in speech pathology and audiology at Marquette University received.

Unfortunately, the students' major (profession) wasn't printed on the degree. It isn't routinely printed on bachelor's degrees at Marquette University. Because of this, some potential employers didn't accept their degree certificate as evidence of professional competence. This necessitated a great deal of letter writing. Consequently, we'd recommend that anybody conducting a professional training program in a developing country for which a degree is awarded arrange to have the name of the profession printed on the degree, even if this isn't customary at their institution.

THE GRADUATION CEREMONY

A traditional Marquette University graduation ceremony was held in Gaza City in July, 1996. The students wore caps and gowns and there was an academic procession. The ceremony was conducted by Dr. Frances Lazarus, Vice President for Academic Affairs at Marquette University. President Yasser Arafat was to be the commencement speaker, but had to make an emergency trip to Egypt about an hour before the ceremony. Both President Arafat's "Personal Representative" and the Minister of Health for the Palestinian Authority filled in for him.

The booklet distributed to persons attending the ceremony was the same one distributed at Marquette University's May, 1996 graduation ceremony. We decided to include the names of the graduates of our program in this booklet (listed alphabetically with those on campus who received B.S. degrees with majors in speech pathology and audiology) to communicate to the students, their families, and others attending the ceremony that their degree was a regular Marquette University one.

In addition to awarding Bachelor of Science degrees to each of the 33 graduates of the program, Marquette University at the ceremony awarded an honorary Doctor of Laws degree to Dr. Hatem Abu-Ghazaleh (see Appendix F for the citation that accompanied this degree).

MEETING POST-GRADUATION RESPONSIBILITIES

For most of the short-term and long-term faculty, their contact (mostly via e-mail and fax) with at least a few of the graduates went beyond (in some cases considerably beyond) what was usual for them—i.e., writing letters of recommendation for graduate schools and/or jobs. One, for example, brought a graduate of the Program to the United States and allowed him to live for a while in his home. Another convinced a United States Senator to help straighten out a credentialing problem that a graduate was having with our State Department. And many offered at least one of the graduates professional advice and support on an ongoing basis.

The continued involvement of the faculty with the graduates wasn't entirely altruistic. The uniqueness of both the Program and the environment in Gaza caused many to bond with these students more closely than they usually did with ones on their campus. In fact, they may have bonded to the extent of becoming an honorary aunt or uncle to at least one of them or possibly even an honorary father or mother.

Chapter 5
Impacts on Students

A necessary task when evaluating any program is to *partially* document the impacts—both positive and negative—that participating in it has had, to date, on those who did so. Such documentation, of course, can never be complete because it isn't possible to completely document anything (Johnson, 1946). There is always more that could be said.

Such documentation can, also, never be completely error free. Regardless of the methodology used to assess the impacts of a program, there are several sources from which error can arise. One such source is never being able to know for certain what would have happened to a participant if he or she hadn't participated. In the context of our program, it isn't possible to know for certain whether something that happened to one of our graduates during the past four years would have happened anyway.

Another probable source of error is observer bias. Such bias could arise from our graduates and/or from us. Our graduates may have only reported impacts they considered significant and/or somehow linked to the Program. Consequently, some positive impacts may not have been reported, and/or the Project participants may have wanted to spare our feelings by not reporting some negative ones. Possible sources of observer bias for us would be failing to delve into all the areas that could have been affected by the Program (e.g., "subconsciously" avoiding ones in which the graduates could have been affected negatively) and/or filtering the data in ways that would be likely to cast the best possible light on the Project.

Yet another possible source of error for the outcome data reported in this chapter is being unable to contact all of the graduates. We had to rely on e-mail and fax to do so and were only successful in getting usable outcome information from about half of them.

Because of the possible sources of error described above and our inability to get outcome data from all of our graduates, the conclusions reported in this chapter should be regarded as tentative. Then too, it takes far longer than four years after graduation to even come close to fully documenting the impacts of any program on its graduates. This is particularly true for this Project because the ongoing conflict (Intifada) between Israelis and Palestinians in the Gaza Strip has produced an economy there that impeded the ability of its graduates to benefit maximally from the training program and the bachelor's degree, either professionally or otherwise.

DID THE STUDENTS BENEFIT SIGNIFICANTLY TO DATE FROM PARTICIPATING IN THE PROGRAM?

The answer to this question is, of course, subjective. What one person would regard as being a significant benefit would not necessarily be so regarded by another. And a person receiving a benefit and those who evaluate its impact on him or her may not agree on whether the amount of impact that it had was significant. That said, it seems clear to us that almost all (perhaps all) of the students benefited significantly from their participation in the Program and almost all of them have informally acknowledged such to us. However, the assumed and/or reported benefits (some of which are described in the next section) were not the same for all participants. Then too, some of the benefits reported may not have been expected by those who designed the Project.

IN WHAT SPECIFIC WAYS DID THE STUDENTS BENEFIT TO DATE FROM PARTICIPATING IN THE PROGRAM?

Judging from feedback from students and faculty over the past five years, the Project's impact has been positive. Some of the ways that students have benefited are indicated in this section. The order in which they're dealt with isn't intended to be significant.

Having a University Degree

Palestinian parents, particularly ones residing in refugee camps, value higher education. There are undoubtedly a number of reasons. Perhaps one is that it's likely to make it possible for their children to get higher paying jobs than they would otherwise and, consequently, be in a better position to help support their family (see student comments in Chapter 3). Comments from our graduates indicate that, as a result of their training and college degree, many are better able to care for themselves and their families. Those that have not yet benefited to the extent that they had hoped remain optimistic for a brighter future. Being able to help support their family would tend to increase their parents and/or siblings respect for them and, consequently, would benefit them.

Having a Degree from a Foreign University

Judging by comments made to us by our students (see student comments in Chapter 3) and a number of persons with whom we spoke in Gaza, it would appear that most Gazans considered degrees from the local universities to be less prestigious than those from foreign institutions of higher education. And among degrees from foreign universities, those from the U.S. appeared to be the most prestigious. In this regard, one of the students commented that the program "offered an education with such high standards that it caused most students in the local universities to envy us."

Gaining a Kind of Citizen-Like Status

Our students, even those who didn't live in refugee camps, weren't citizens of any country. Their country, Palestine, no longer existed. Their status, as Palestinians, in Israel and its Territories (the Gaza Strip and the West Bank) was that of *alien*, as it was in Arab Countries (except for Jordan) and elsewhere (Said, 1986). Their receipt of a degree from an American university conferred on them a kind of international citizenship. That is, it made them citizens of the international community of scholars. This "citizenship" has, for example, facilitated several of them being admitted to universities in other countries (including the United States, England, and Canada) for graduate study.

Getting a Job as a Speech-Language Pathologist, Audiologist, or Teacher of the Deaf

It was hoped that, when the students graduated, the economy in the Gaza Strip would be good enough for all of them to find employment there as speech-language pathologists, audiologists, or teachers of the deaf. Unfortunately, only about a third of them were able to do so. One, incidentally, did do so in the United Arab Emirates.

Hopefully, the economy in the Gaza Strip will improve sufficiently to enable more of the Project graduates to find employment specific to their training. It's worth noting, however, that even though some of the graduates have not yet found employment in the fields of communication disorders and special education, most have been able to use their degrees as a means of obtaining respectable employment. Recalling that the unemployment rate in the Gaza Strip was close to 100 percent for women and 50 percent for men during the past five years, the ability of almost all our graduates who remained there to find respectable employment is impressive.

Even if the economy in the Gaza Strip were to improve sufficiently for all of our graduates to be employed there in one of these fields, it is doubtful that all of them would be interested in having such a job. At least a few of them were (or became) more interested in other fields. One of our graduates, for example, began a masters degree program in Administrative Science and Developmental Problems in the Department of Politics at a university in England (York University) about a year after graduating.

Getting Another Kind of Job Because of Having a University Degree

Most of the students who remained in the Gaza Strip and were unable to find employment there as speech-language pathologists, audiologists, or teachers of the deaf did get a relatively well-paying job (by Gazan standards) because of having a university degree and some proficiency with English. A number of our graduates were employed by the United Nations Relief and Works Agency (UNRWA), which had moved at least some of its administrative offices to the Gaza Strip.

Having a Better Standard of Living Than Previously

Almost all of the students who were not pursuing graduate degrees reported that their standard of living was considerably better than it had been prior to graduating. Some of them were even secure enough financially to purchase cars.

Being Better Able to Assist One's Family, Financially and Otherwise

Many of the students assisted their families financially after graduating. There may have been a greater need than previously for them to do so: If their fathers and/or siblings had worked in Israel, they may have lost their jobs because the political situation and/or the Intifada caused the border between the Gaza Strip and Israel to be closed.

They may have also been able to assist their families by increasing their status within the Palestinian community. Just as a lower socio-economic family in the United States would be likely to gain some status by having a son or daughter graduate from an "Ivy League" university, a Palestinian family would be likely to gain some special status by having a son or daughter graduate from an American university.

Becoming More Proficient with English

While the courses that the students took in English-as-a-second-language were only intended to be a means to an end—i.e., to make it possible for the instruction to be in English—they turned out to be a significant benefit for the students. That is, the resulting improvement in English enhanced their opportunities for both employment and graduate study. They also enhanced their ability to utilize the Internet for both e-mail communication and securing needed information.

At the end of the Program, the students varied considerably in their ability to understand, speak, read, and write English (particularly the latter). All of them had become more proficient with it, sufficiently so to earn at least the minimum GPA needed for graduation. Yet some, even at graduation, probably couldn't pass the English competency examination that many American universities require foreign students to pass as a condition for admission. In a sense, our graduates were like the bumblebees who, so said some early engineers, weren't designed for flight but, not knowing this, flew anyway.

Becoming Computer-Literate

Students spent many hours using state-of-the-art PCs for word processing (e.g., clinical report writing) and other applications (e.g., audiometric testing). They had access to PCs at a computer lab in the classroom building and at the audiology and speech clinics. One evidence of their having become computer literate is that most had acquired an e-mail address within two years after graduating.

Becoming Better Able to Think and Reason Maturely

One of the goals of the liberal arts component of Marquette University's undergraduate programs is to facilitate students' abilities to think and reason maturely.

Judging by both comments that the students made to us and our observations of their behavior, the ability of most of them to do so increased significantly during the period they were in the Program.

Being More Respected Than Previously

The fact that the students now had a university degree (particularly one from an American University) would be expected to result in their being more highly respected that previously, by Palestinians and by others.

Having a Better Self-Concept

A number of the students commented that their participation in the Program caused them to feel better about themselves. The reason undoubtedly was, in part, earning a university degree. But it may also have been related to surviving an "Outward Bound" type of experience. That is, they completed the requirements for their degree under extraordinarily difficult circumstances, which included having to cope with such things as the Israeli occupation, the Intifada, general strikes called by Hamas that they had to violate (at risk of injury) to attend class, and extreme poverty.

Pursuing Graduate Study

At least six of the students, when this chapter was written, were working on or had received a masters degree from a university in the United States, England, Canada, or Jordan. Several others have indicated to us that they hope to be able to seek a graduate degree. With possibly one or two exceptions, we felt that the students had both the motivation and ability to complete a masters degree program. Many, in fact, probably have the ability to complete a Ph.D. It is our hope (which we've communicated to a number of the students) that at least half a dozen of them will eventually get a Ph.D. and establish a department in a Palestinian University that will offer majors in speech-language pathology, audiology, and deaf education.

Being Able to Leave the Gaza Strip

Considering the violence, economic and political problems, and the lack of opportunities for Palestinians in the Gaza Strip, it isn't particularly surprising that several of the students wanted desperately to leave and did. Obviously, having a university degree (particularly one from an American university) made it easier for them to do so. Hopefully, this "brain drain" will not be permanent.

Learning to Interact with Peers of the Opposite Sex

It is traditional in Moslem countries for males and females to be educated separately. We were told that our program was the first in the Gaza Strip in which both sexes attended class together. It would have been impractical for use to teach them separately. Attending class with members of the opposite sex did initially appear to make some of the students feel uncomfortable. However, almost all of the students adjusted quickly to the situation and learned to interact with each other appropriately as classmates.

Being Able to Marry Outside of the Family

It is traditional in the Gaza Strip both for marriages to be arranged and for many of them to be between first cousins. Several of the students fell in love with classmates and married them. A few of the students, incidentally, commented to us that they didn't want an arranged marriage with first cousins because they didn't want their children to be at greater than usual risk for having genetic deformities.

Acquiring New Friendships and Networking Possibilities

The students developed friendships with classmates and with the faculty who participated in the Program. Many of them were still in relatively frequent e-mail and snail mail contact with both fellow students and faculty when this chapter was written. The students also founded the Palestinian Speech and Hearing Association, in part, as a vehicle for networking among themselves and possibly also internationally.

Being in a Better Position to Assume a Leadership Role in the Palestinian Territories

Having a bachelor's degree, particularly one from an American university, would be expected to put our graduates in a better position to assume leadership roles. Those who went on to get graduate degrees would, of course, be in even a better position to do so. The leadership roles they assume could extend beyond helping persons who are communicatively impaired.

Gaining Greater Ability "to be a Person for Others"

One aspect of Marquette University's Jesuit tradition is to encourage its graduates, even ones who aren't Catholics, "to be persons for others." Most of our students at the beginning of the Program appeared to have the inclination to be so. Through the training they received in communicative disorders and their exposure to the liberal arts core, their ability to actualize their potential to do so was enhanced.

IN WHAT WAYS MIGHT STUDENTS HAVE BEEN HARMED TO DATE BY PARTICIPATING IN THE PROGRAM?

We are only aware of two possible ways that students may have been harmed by participating in our program. The first is that one of them went to England and died unexpectedly while working on a master's degree. He probably wouldn't have been in England if he hadn't graduated from our program. We are uncertain about the circumstances of his death and the extent to which they were related to his being there.

The second way that students may have been harmed by participating is by being unable to achieve employment-related goals. The students expected that they would have a job in the Gaza Strip as a speech-language pathologist, audiologist, or teacher of the deaf after graduating. This expectation was not unrealistic. They were required to sign an agreement to be accepted into the Program that obligated them to work in the Gaza Strip in one of these professions for several years after graduating. Furthermore, they all knew that the purpose of the Project (and the reason for it being funded by USAID) was to provide clinicians and teachers to meet the rehabilitation and educational needs of persons in the Gaza Strip who had a speech, language, and/or hearing impairment. Unfortunately, the funding that the Palestinian Authority and the Society for the Care of the Handicapped in the Gaza Strip had available for rehabilitation and special education when they graduated wasn't sufficient to provide jobs for all of them. Nevertheless, almost all of those who were unable to get a job in the Gaza Strip in one of these fields were able to get one there in another because of having a bachelor's degree.

HOW DO THE GRADUATES HOPE TO BENEFIT IN THE FUTURE FROM THEIR PARTICIPATION IN THE PROGRAM?

Almost all of our graduates hope to eventually be able to work in the Gaza Strip as speech-language pathologists, audiologists, or teachers of the deaf. Some of those who were unable to find employment in Gaza in one of these fields were involved, at least marginally, in the founding and nurturing of the Palestinian Speech and Hearing Association. Furthermore, a few of the graduates (who have sufficiently strong family ties to Gaza to be unlikely to contribute to its "brain drain") were abroad working on graduate degrees in one of these fields when this chapter was written.

All of our graduates, of course, also want what college graduates everywhere want—i.e., an economically secure future for themselves and their families. While almost all of them are more secure economically now than they were prior to graduating, they have a long way to go before they'll be able to insure themselves and their families of such a future.

IF THE GRADUATES KNEW IN 1992 WHAT THEY KNOW NOW ABOUT THE PROGRAM AND ITS IMPACTS, WOULD THEY STILL HAVE PARTICIPATED IN IT?

While we didn't ask the students this question directly, judging by comments they've made to us (e.g., see the student comments in Chapter 3) we suspect that almost all—perhaps all—of them would answer "Yes."

Chapter 6

Impacts on Communicatively-Handicapped Persons and Their Families

The primary purpose of the Project was to generate rehabilitation and educational services for the tens of thousands of children and adults in the Gaza Strip who were speech, language, and/or hearing impaired. It was not to better the lives of the 33 graduates of our training program, though we certainly did hope that their lives would be better than they would've been otherwise (see Chapter 5 for information about the impacts of the Project on them). Consequently, it is both appropriate and necessary in an evaluation of this project to consider its impacts on the communicatively-impaired children and adults who resided in the Gaza Strip, as well as the impact the project had on their families. These impacts are dealt with in this chapter.

DID THE PROJECT RESULT IN MORE SERVICES BEING AVAILABLE TO COMMUNICATIVELY-IMPAIRED PEOPLE LIVING WITHIN THE GAZA STRIP?

More communicatively-impaired children and adults in the Gaza Strip received rehabilitation and educational services as a result of this project than undoubtedly would have been the case otherwise. With the exception of a small, privately-funded school for the deaf, no entity in the Gaza Strip other than the Society for the Care of the Handicapped offered such services while the Project was ongoing. Few of those who received services through the Project could have afforded to get them elsewhere.

More than fifteen hundred communicatively-impaired children and adults received such services from the Society for the Care of the Handicapped while the Project was ongoing. Initially the students observed diagnostic, teaching, and therapeutic services being provided and then increasingly participated in providing them. The goal was to get the students competent to provide these services, without supervision, after the Project terminated. It was also hoped that program graduates would, at some point, be proficient and professional enough to be able to train future generations of audiologists, speech-language pathologists, and teachers of deaf children.

Services for persons who were speech and/or hearing impaired continued to be available to residents of Gaza after the Project terminated, but were not as easily accessible as previously. There were at least two reasons, both of which were funding related. The first was fewer personnel. Funding wasn't available to hire all of our graduates after the training project ended. The second was the loss of subsidies for services. During the Project, clinical and teaching fees were subsidized by the grant such that costs to the Palestinians were minimal. With the end of the USAID funding, charges for services had to be sufficient to at least cover costs. In too many cases, this made the services too expensive, particularly for those who needed hearing aids or long-term therapy.

WHAT TYPES OF REHABILITATION AND EDUCATIONAL SERVICES WHERE PROVIDED BY THE PROJECT WHILE IT WAS ONGOING?

Perhaps because the facilities for audiological services were fully operational before those for deaf education and speech-language pathology, the Project was more noted for audiological services such as hearing testing and hearing aid fitting. However, several hundred deaf children did receive educational services through the Society's home-based program for preschoolers and its classroom-based program for school-age children. And more than a hundred children who had a speech or language disorder that wasn't caused by a hearing loss received therapy. The causes of their disorders included mental retardation, autism, cleft palate, cerebral palsy, head injury, psychological trauma, and faulty learning. Some of the head injury cases, even in preschoolers, resulted from gun shot wounds that were acquired during the Intifada.

WHAT KINDS OF IMPACTS DID THESE SERVICES HAVE ON THE PERSONS WHO RECEIVED THEM?

These services impacted on those who received them in several ways. For some it reduced the severity of or eliminated their impairment. For example, the hearing aids that those who were hard-of-hearing received reduced the severity of the impact of their impairment. And many of the children who had articulation or language disorders caused by faulty learning were cured.

For many of those whose impairment couldn't be eliminated, the rehabilitation and educational services provided reduced significantly the disability and handicap that did (or could in the future) result from it. For example, the educational and rehabilitation services that most of the children who were deaf received reduced significantly the severity of the disability resulting from their impairment, thereby causing them to be less handicapped than they probably would have been otherwise. The same was true for hard-of-hearing persons whose impairment could not be eliminated by hearing aids and for those with speech or language impairments who could not be cured.

WHAT IMPACTS DID THESE SERVICES HAVE ON THE FAMILIES OF PERSONS WHO RECEIVED THEM?

Palestinians tend to care deeply about their families. Consequently, a family member's handicapping condition causes great concern. It follows, then, that services which ameliorated the negative impact of handicapping conditions were much appreciated by the Palestinian people.

WHAT KINDS OF IMPACTS DID THESE SERVICES HAVE ON PERSONS IN THE GAZA STRIP WHO DID NOT RECEIVE THEM?

Only a relatively small percentage of the persons in the Gaza Strip with significant hearing, speech, or language impairments received services while the Program was ongoing. It, nevertheless, in all likelihood impacted on others and/or their families. Several ways that it may have done so are indicated in this section.

Alerted Them to the Existence of Such Services and What It Is Possible for Them to Accomplish

In developed countries, including the United States, there are many persons (including health-care professionals) who are not aware of the range of services that speech-language pathologists, audiologists, and deaf educators provide and what it is possible for such services to accomplish. Not unexpectedly, it is too often the case that the residents of developing countries are not aware of the potential benefits of such services. How did the people living in the Gaza Strip learn about the services offered through the Project? Through the local media, through word-of-mouth, and through our students who helped to spread the good news.

Modified their Attitudes Toward and Expectations for Persons Who Have a Hearing, Speech, and/or Language Impairment

Negative attitudes toward and low expectations for those having impairments often contribute to the disability and/or handicap they yield. Such attitudes and expectations exist throughout the world. While we didn't systematically evaluate in Gaza for changes in attitudes and expectations, there is at least a little reason to believe that our program may have facilitated something positive for both.

Possibly Modified Their Conception of "the Will of God" for Treating Such Impairments

Most residents of the Gaza Strip were Moslems and believed that:

> Those who abided strictly by the revelations Mohammed received while in a trance from the angel Gabriel would be rewarded with a "perfect" life. There would be no need to question. Every event, every turn of fortune, would be determined by God. *Inshallah* (If Allah wills it.) Tell an Arab friend that you will see him tomorrow or wish him a safe journey or say that you hope his business meeting goes well, and the reply is always the same— "*Inshallah.*" (Lamb, p. 6)

This "fatalism" can impact either positively or negatively on attitudes toward treating such impairments. If an impairment is viewed as being the "will of God," than attempts to treat it could be considered contrary to God's will. On the other hand, if treatments for the impairment are viewed as being from God, then the "will of God" would be to take advantage of them. As specialists in special education and rehabilitation who aren't Moslems, we consider it more desirable for the view to be the latter than the former. And while we didn't do any surveying about this, we suspect that at least a few residents of Gaza who previously had the former view now have the latter.

WHAT IS THE PROJECT'S SERVICE LEGACY IN THE GAZA STRIP?

As we've indicated previously, some of our graduates offered audiological, speech-language pathology, and deaf education services on a fee-for-service basis utilizing the facilities of the Society for the Care of the Handicapped in the Gaza Strip and those of other disability-related societies in Gaza.

WHAT WILL BE THE PROJECT'S LONG-TERM LEGACY IN THE PALESTINIAN TERRITORIES?

Hopefully, the Project's long-term legacy in the Gaza Strip and West Bank will include the following:

- An increased awareness among special education and rehabilitation specialists in these territories (and hopefully also among the general public in them) that it's possible to treat hearing, speech, and language impairments and by so doing, reduce the severity of the disabilities and handicaps that they tend to produce.
- A reduction in the incidence of certain communicative impairments (e.g., deafness and stuttering) because of greater awareness of what can be done to prevent them or reduce the likelihood of their occurrence.
- More rehabilitation and educational services for children and adults who have a hearing, speech, and/or language impairment.
- A bachelor's or master's degree major in communicative disorders at a Palestinian university. Such a program could be, at least partially, staffed by graduates of our program, particularly ones who have gotten master's degrees. Even if all of the graduates of our program worked professionally in the Palestinian territories, they would be too few to meet the need.

WHAT CAN BE DONE BY NON-GOVERNMENT ORGANIZATIONS (NGOS) AND OTHERS TO PROMOTE THE DEVELOPMENT OF SERVICES FOR PERSONS IN THE GAZA STRIP AND WEST BANK WHO ARE COMMUNICATIVELY IMPAIRED?

As long as it is necessary for rehabilitation and special educational services for persons in the Palestinian territories who have a hearing, speech, or language impairment to be offered on a fee-for-service basis, many will not receive them because they or their families can't afford them. It's difficult to visualize a scenario in the foreseeable future that would result in the economy in the Palestinian territories improving sufficiently for a subsidy for such services being unnecessary. Hopefully, at least one NGO will be motivated in the near future (perhaps, in part, by this book) to subsidize disability-related societies in the West Bank and Gaza Strip to provide these services.

Chapter 7
Impacts on Participating Faculty and Institutions

To be deemed a success, our training program had to positively impact the 33 participating students and it had to benefit the communicatively-handicapped people living in the Gaza Strip. Though it is too early to conclude that the program will become a long-term success, we can say that the initial goals of the Project have been met (see Chapters 5 and 6).

Two other groups on whom we felt it worthwhile to try to evaluate the impact of the Project were the faculty who participated in the program and their universities. While the project was not designed to impact positively on participating faculty, we felt that it probably did so judging by the fact that almost all of them after returning from Gaza told us that they would welcome the opportunity to teach there again or in another developing country. There is also some reason to believe that it impacted positively on their universities. Some impacts that participating may have had on both are indicated in this chapter.

POSSIBLE IMPACTS ON PARTICIPATING FACULTY

Gaining a More Objective Attitude Toward Palestinians

A number of participating faculty after returning from Gaza commented to us that their attitude toward Palestinians was more positive than it had been previously. This change was undoubted due in large part to getting to know the students and other Palestinians as people. It also, for at least some, appeared to have been due to hearing about, observing, and experiencing how some members of the Israeli

Defense Force (IDF) and some Israeli airport security personnel tend to treat both Palestinians and internationals (like themselves) who interact with them.

Deriving Pleasure from Helping Those Considered Less Fortunate

If you've volunteered to help somebody whom you considered less fortunate than you and the help was appreciated, you're likely to be familiar with the pleasure that can be derived from doing so. The students communicated to the faculty by both "word and deed" how much they appreciated their coming to Gaza to teach them and most continued doing so (to some of them) after they graduated.

Having Students Who Are Truly Interested in What You Teach

Many of the Marquette University faculty who taught liberal arts core courses commented that it was a real pleasure teaching these students because most of them (unlike most of those whom they taught on campus who weren't liberal arts majors) seemed to be really interested in and excited by the subject matter.

Accepting a Challenge That's Widely Regarded as Being Risky

Doing so is likely to enhance one's self-concept. Some people, for example, take up sky diving for this reason. Information in the media (e.g., CNN) throughout the four year period that the Project was ongoing suggested that the Gaza Strip was a dangerous place to be. Consequently, most of those who went probably regarded themselves as accepting a challenge that was at least a little risky. Their friends and family probably did also and viewed their willingness to risk to help handicapped children as being commendable (which, of course, if communicated to them could contribute to enhancing their self-concepts).

Enhancing One's Reputation Locally, Nationally, and Internationally

Some of those who taught in the program became more widely known and respected locally, nationally, and/or internationally because of doing so. Stories about the Project and their participation in it appeared in local media; they gave talks about it to the general public; they gave presentations on it to local, national, and international professional groups; and they wrote articles about it for professional journals and newsletters.

Reducing the Likelihood of "Burnout"

The professional life of many academics after a number of years becomes routine. Consequently, it offers less intellectual stimulation than previously and can cause them to "burn out." One way that an academic can reduce the likelihood of it happening is to do something different professionally. Short-term teaching in Gaza undoubtedly helped some (including both of us) to delay burning out.

Traveling Internationally at Somebody Else's Expense

Teaching in the program gave participating faculty an opportunity to travel internationally at little cost to themselves. While the intensiveness of the program left little time for sightseeing, almost all got to spend at least one day visiting such places as Jerusalem, Bethlehem, and Tel Aviv.

Learning at a "Gut Level" about Another Culture

Participating faculty lived among Palestinians and interacted with them daily. Our faculty, like other residents of Gaza, had to cope with nightly curfews, general strikes, purposeful cutoffs of electricity, travel restrictions, and other indignities. But our faculty also experienced the extraordinary hospitality and warmth so characteristic of the Palestinian people. Some of our faculty, in fact, became honorary members of Palestinian families.

Income

Participating faculty received a salary that more than covered their out-of-pocket expenses for the trip, including sightseeing, restaurant meals, and souvenirs (e.g., hand-woven rugs). Since most of the faculty were under long-term contracts with their home universities during the time they taught for us, their pay from their regular positions continued even as they were being paid for their services in Gaza. They were, then, "double dipping" and most took home a sizable check. It must be noted, however, that some of the Marquette faculty returned their salaries to the Project—donating their salaries back to the Palestinian people.

Convention Presentations and Publications

Some participants (including both authors) did convention presentations and/or published articles about the Project and their participation in it.

Increased Visibility to Upper Administration

Some of the participants from Marquette and Lamar Universities got to interact with (and consequently, became better known to) persons in their home university's upper administration (e.g., their Vice President for Academic Affairs and/or President) with whom they probably would have had little or no contact otherwise. This "visibility" could yield them some protection at the local level (department and college) because of it being assumed there that they have upper administrative support. Furthermore, it could result in their talents being recognized by upper administration and, consequently, be career enhancing.

New Friendships and Interests

Many of the friendships that faculty formed with others who taught in the program and with students and other Palestinians they met while in Gaza were maintained after they returned to the States. The networking that resulted has yielded a number of opportunities, including chances to lecture internationally.

Most of the participants returned to the states considerably more interested in Palestinians and the Israeli-Palestinian peace process than they were previously. Furthermore, almost all were hoping to have more opportunities to do short-term lecturing and/or teaching internationally.

Religious Conversion

One of the teachers of English as a second language became a Moslem.

POSSIBLE IMPACTS ON PARTICIPATING UNIVERSITIES

Enhancing the Institution's Image Locally, Nationally, and Internationally

Articles about the Project and some of those who participated in it appeared in the Marquette and Lamar University student newspaper, faculty/staff newsletter, and alumni magazine. They also appeared in local newspapers and in state, national, and international professional publications. Since the ultimate purpose of the Project was to help handicapped children, the image of both institutions even appeared to be enhanced in the American Jewish community and in Israel. With regard to the latter, several presentations about the Project were given in Israel* and several organizations within Israel expressed interest in partially replicating it.**

Attracting (Recruiting) Students—Both Nationals and Internationals

Both Marquette University and Lamar University recruited at least a few students from the Gaza Strip as a direct result of their participation in the Project. Dr. Hatem Abu Ghazaleh's youngest son, for example, went to Marquette University for his Bachelor's degree. And one of our audiology graduates went to Lamar University on a Fulbright Fellowship for a masters degree.

Establishing Mutually-Beneficial Relationships with Foreign GOs and NGOs

Both universities have directly established good relationships with individuals within the Palestinian National Authority and the Society for the Care of the Handicapped in the Gaza Strip. They have also indirectly established such relationships with some of the other organizations in the Palestinian Territories who employed our graduates. While they haven't made positive use of these relationships yet (to our knowledge), they may do so in the future.

Increasing Opportunities for Their Faculty to Function Internationally

Participation in this project has directly or indirectly yielded new opportunities for at least a few of their faculty (including both authors) to function internationally.

Increasing Access to Grant Funding

Participation in the Project made both institutions subcontractors in the USAID grant that funded it. Furthermore, the visibility and good will that both gained in the Moslem community (nationally and internationally) through their involvement with this project which helped handicapped Moslem children has the potential to increase their viability for grant funding from foundations in this community.

---

* One was at the Eighteenth International Congress on Education of the Deaf, in Tel Aviv in July, 1995.

** These included the 'Eden' Association, which is based in Kibbutz Shoval in the Northern Negev.

POSSIBLE IMPACTS ON PALESTINIANS OTHER THAN ONES ON PROJECT PARTICIPANTS AND ON THE AREA'S COMMUNICATIVELY HANDICAPPED

Employment Opportunities

The Society for the Care of the Handicapped was one of the five largest employers in the Gaza Strip. At least 350 of its employees received all or part of their salary from the USAID grant for the Project.

Increased Availability of Needed Staff

The program provided audiologists, speech-language pathologists, and teachers of the deaf for a number of rehabilitation and special education facilities in the Gaza Strip. There were no audiologists or speech-language pathologists and very few teachers of the deaf in the Gaza Strip prior to 1992.

More Objective Attitude Toward Americans

A widely-held belief among the people we worked with in Gaza was that Americans were pro Israeli and biased against Palestinians. Our sense is that, just as our faculty's view of Palestinians changed during the course of the Project, so too did the Palestinian's opinion of Americans change because of the Project. We were told again and again how much the Palestinian people appreciated the financial support from USAID, how much they liked the fact that our faculty treated them with respect, and how pleased they were that we were training their young people for entry into a profession that would improve the lives of the handicapped people of the Gaza Strip. In this regard, a speaker at the banquet the Palestinian Authority had for participants in the Project after the graduation ceremony (July, 1996) commented that President Arafat and others in the Palestinian Authority considered this program to be strong evidence that at least some Americans really cared about Palestinians.

More Objective Attitude Toward Jews

One of us (FHS) is Jewish. Prior to 1994, the only Jews whom many of the students and staff at the Society had encountered were either members of the Israeli Defense Force (IDF) or employers in Israel. Our students were not usually treated respectfully by either. In fact, many of the Project participants had served time in Israeli prisons. The students and many of the staff of the Society knew that FHS was Jewish and most (if not all) appeared to feel that they were treated respectfully by him. Comments made by students and members of the staff at the Society suggest that they had modified their attitude toward Jews to the extent of being willing to at least consider the possibility that "some are okay."

Enhancement of Image Internationally

Information about the Project appeared in publications for both professionals and the general public in the United States and elsewhere. It undoubtedly contributed to making a little more positive the negative stereotype for Palestinians held by at least a few persons internationally.

Chapter 8
Implications for Training Rehabilitation and Special Education Professionals in Developing Countries

In previous chapters, the Project was viewed from the perspective of its intended purpose (goal) which was to meet a practical need—i.e., to provide personnel to help children and adults in the Gaza Strip who are communicatively impaired. We will be viewing it in this chapter from a different perspective—as an experiment intended to test the effectiveness of certain strategies for training rehabilitation and special education professionals in developing countries. Doing so results in both the students and participating faculty being considered research subjects. While what we learned by viewing them in this way is, of course, most applicable to training audiologists, speech-language pathologists, and teachers of the deaf, much (perhaps almost all) of it is also applicable to training professionals in other rehabilitation and special education fields.

The data we gathered, though anecdotal, provides at least partial answers to a number of questions. Some of these will be dealt with in this chapter. The order in which they're dealt with isn't intended to suggest their importance or anything else.

IS THE GOAL OF INITIALLY TRAINING REHABILITATION OR SPECIAL EDUCATION PRACTITIONERS ON A PROFESSIONAL (RATHER THAN ON A TECHNICIAN) LEVEL FOR A DEVELOPING COUNTRY ACHIEVABLE?

We were successful in training rehabilitation practitioners (audiologists and speech-language pathologists) and special education teachers (teachers of the deaf) to function at a level at, or close, to that for professionals in these fields in the United States. Consequently, we conclude that this goal is achievable in a developing country.

While the goal of initially training practitioners in a developing country to function as professionals is apparently achievable, is it desirable? That is, would it be better to begin by training lower functioning practitioners (i.e., technicians) instead of fully-trained professionals? The main advantage of training them at the technician level would be that it would take less time to do so. And because it would take less time to train them, those trained would be available sooner to help persons who could benefit from their services.

Perhaps the main disadvantage to training technicians at the onset is that, lacking advanced training, technicians need levels of supervision that are probably not available in a developing country. And they're going to have to function independentally if they're to continue to function effectively after they graduate unless you can arrange for somebody to be there permanently to supervise them. This, of course, is a commitment that you're unlikely to be able to make.

Another disadvantage faced by technicians is that, lacking a bachelor's degree, they have fewer opportunities to upgrade themselves professionally. If they have a bachelor's degree from a college or university that's accredited and respected internationally, they might be eligible to do graduate work in a developed country (assuming that their GPA is sufficiently high) and to apply for the financial aid they'll probably need. Two of our graduates are now doing graduate work, one in the U.S. and one in England. Both have earned prestigious competitive fellowships. A third completed a graduate degree in England and began a second but, sadly, died before competing the second graduate degree.

Compared to fully-trained professionals, technicians in a developing country are less likely to be afforded the respect they need to develop their professional field. It seems a poor decision now, but when the program was initiated, the intent was to train technicians and to award program graduates a certificate of completion. After thinking this through, it was decided to upgrade the program—to award a bachelor's degree. For this reason, Marquette University was invited to join the Project to teach the liberal arts component and to award the undergraduate degree.

IS IT PRACTICAL TO BRING THE TRAINING PROGRAM TO THE STUDENTS?

The fact that we were successful in conducting a bachelor's degree program in Gaza indicates that it's both possible and practical to do this in a developing country. Furthermore, the fact that earlier the University of Calgary did so successfully there also (Brown, Ghazaleh, & Neufeldt, 1996) provides additional support for this conclusion. Using current distance learning technology for some courses, incidentally, could make doing so even more practical.

WHY MIGHT IT BE ADVANTAGEOUS TO BRING THE TRAINING PROGRAM TO THE STUDENTS?

There are several reasons why it's likely to be advantageous to train practitioners in rehabilitation and special education for a developing country in the environment in which they'll be working. First, they'll probably be better able to cope with this environment after graduating if they get some experience doing so before graduating. The knowledge and skills required to function successfully as a practitioner in rehabilitation or special education in a developing country are not identical to those required to do so in a developed country. Less technology and funding, for example, are likely to be available for such services in a developing country than in a developed one. Furthermore, cultural expectations for delivery of such services in a developing country are likely to differ, at least a little, from those in any developed one.

Another reason why it's likely to be advantageous to train practitioners in rehabilitation and special education for a developing country on site is that doing so probably will reduce "brain drain." More persons from a developing country are likely to remain "at home" after graduating if they are trained there. Possible reasons for persons trained in a developed country not returning include acquiring a spouse or "significant other," being able to practice with less hassle, and being able to have a higher standard of living.

HOW DO YOU RECRUIT FACULTY TO TEACH SHORT-TERM IN A DEVELOPING COUNTRY?

If our experience is representative, recruiting faculty to teach short-term in a war-torn developing country is difficult, particularly in the early stage of a project. Recruiting is likely to become less difficult after the first few faculty return because many (perhaps most) persons who do such teaching find it very rewarding—perhaps the most rewarding teaching they've ever done. Almost all of our short-term faculty, incidentally, either returned to Gaza to teach additional courses or expressed an interest in doing so.

Perhaps the key to success to recruiting short-term faculty for such a project is having one or more upper university administrators who are strongly committed to the project and, consequently, highly motivated to do whatever is necessary (so long as it is both legal and ethical) to actively recruit faculty. There were two such administrators involved with this project: Dr. Frances Lazarus, who was Marquette University's Vice President for Academic Affairs, and one of us (RM), who was Lamar University's Graduate College Dean and Associate Vice President for Research.

To begin to recruit faculty from Marquette University to teach the 18-course liberal arts core, Dr. Lazarus held informal informational meetings. He invited FHS, who had already taught several courses in Gaza, to provide a description of the Project, describe life in the Gaza Strip, and candidly answer questions. Dr. Lazarus also met individually with faculty whom he thought were viable for teaching in Gaza and did what he could to motivate them to participate. When the first few faculty returned to Marquette, they were quite vocal and enthusiastic about their experience and, consequently, recruitment became somewhat less difficult.

The original plan called for all of the professional courses to be taught by Lamar University faculty. While a number of Lamar faculty did participate in the program, not enough could be recruited to teach all of the necessary courses. Consequently, it was necessary to secure short-term faculty for the program from other institutions. This was done by placing an advertisement in several national publications specific to communication disorders and deaf education. One of us (FHS), incidentally, became involved with the program by responding to such an advertisement.

WHAT INFORMATION SHOULD BE PROVIDED FACULTY BEFORE THEY TEACH THEIR FIRST COURSE IN A DEVELOPING COUNTRY?

It's desirable for recruitment and other reasons for the experience of teaching in the program to be pleasant overall. New faculty need to be completely briefed on such things as dress, housing, customs, economics, weather, etc. The document in Appendix D can serve as at least a partial model for one intended for this purpose.

IS IT PRACTICAL TO PROVIDE A LIBERAL ARTS UNDERGRADUATE DEGREE IN A DEVELOPING COUNTRY?

The fact that our program was successful is compelling evidence for the practicality of such a training program. However, to succeed, such a program must have enthusiastic students and a committed, quality faculty. Our program was successful, in part, because both the students and the associated local NGO (Society for the Care of the Handicapped in the Gaza Strip) were highly motivated by the bachelor's degree.

IS IT ADVANTAGEOUS FOR A TRAINING PROGRAM LIKE OURS TO HAVE A LIBERAL ARTS CORE?

There are a number of reasons why it could be advantageous for a training program like ours to have a liberal arts core. Perhaps the most compelling is that such a core helps "...to better prepare people to think, plan, judge, empathize, wonder, hypothesize, criticize, test, invent, and imagine" (Anderson, 1993, p. 3). Consequently, it helps to prepare them to both function independently and assume a leadership role. Both are necessary if the field for which they're being trained is to thrive in their country after they graduate.

IS IT PRACTICAL FOR ALMOST ALL OF THE INSTRUCTION IN A PROGRAM STRUCTURED LIKE OURS TO BE IN ENGLISH?

It's practical for almost all of the instruction to be in English if there is a sufficient number of qualified students available who can communicate well in English. Alternatively, you can admit into your program students whose English skills are somewhat weak if you are willing to expend the time and resources to teach English as a Second Language (ESL). While all 33 of our students had a little knowledge of English before entering the program, few (if any) had English speaking and literacy skills that were adequate for pursuing college-level study.

We provided extensive ESL training and, in our opinion, this training and the experience associated with the English-only lectures and texts culminated in dramatically improved English skills that were at least minimally sufficient for university-level training.

WHY MIGHT IT BE ADVANTAGEOUS FOR ALMOST ALL OF THE INSTRUCTION TO BE IN ENGLISH?

The ability to read books, journals, and Internet material in English is an essential skill for any professional in a developing country if he or she is to keep up-to-date. New information is more likely to be published in English than in any other language. English has, in fact, become the international language for professional and scientific publication. Consequently, "forcing" students in developing countries to acquire a knowledge of English by having instruction be in it has an added benefit. It provides them with an essential tool for keeping up-to-date.

IF THE LANGUAGE OF INSTRUCTION IS TO BE ENGLISH, WHAT LEVEL OF KNOWLEDGE OF ENGLISH SHOULD BE REQUIRED FOR ADMISSION TO THE PROGRAM?

Ideally, the answer would be a knowledge of English adequate for college-level study. However, the pool of such students who'd be interested in your program is likely to be quite small in most developing countries in which the national language isn't English. Certainly, some knowledge of English should be required for admission, along with an agreement (perhaps in the form of a written contract) to become more proficient through enthusiastic participation in the tutoring that's provided.

HOW FEASIBLE IS IT TO TEACH A THREE SEMESTER HOUR COURSE IN THREE TO FOUR WEEKS?

The fact that the 18 liberal arts core courses and most of the professional courses in our program were taught in this manner is compelling evidence that doing so is feasible. However, if a faculty person is used to teaching a particular course over a normal 13-15 week period, then adjustments in the timing of assignments and in examinations will be necessary.

To the best of our knowledge, all course requirements were completed and grades were submitted by short-term faculty before they left Gaza. However, with the current availability of Internet access in most developing countries, it may be both possible and desirable for some course assignments to be submitted to the instructor via e-mail after he or she leaves. We didn't have this option because Internet access wasn't available in the Gaza Strip (at least to us) while our program was ongoing. It is, however, available there now.

It is now commonly the case that entire courses are taught via the Internet. For example, faculty frequently teach distance education courses via WebCT, which is a software package designed to facilitate web-based internet delivery. Often distance education is delivered via a hybrid of face-to-face and web-based internet delivery. If this hybrid distance learning option had been available to us, we would certainly have given it serious consideration, particularly for some of the liberal arts courses.

HOW LARGE A DROP-OUT RATE SHOULD BE ANTICIPATED FOR SUCH A PROGRAM?

A substantial drop-out rate should be anticipated during the first year, particularly if many of the students aren't proficient in English at the beginning of the program, if English is to be the language of instruction, and/or if high standards are to be maintained. The drop-out rate for our program during the first year was more than 50 percent. We had over a hundred students at the beginning of the program. About half of them dropped out in the first few weeks, a few more in the next month or so, and then it held quite steady for the duration of the program. The main reasons why students left the program (voluntarily or involuntarily) during the first year appeared to be a lack of motivation to do what was necessary to become proficient in English and a lack of money. Even though this was a grant-funded program, there were expenses and the poverty rate in Gaza was overwhelming.

SHOULD STUDENTS BE REQUIRED TO COMMIT TO REMAINING IN THEIR HOME COUNTRY AFTER THE COMPLETION OF THE TRAINING PROGRAM?

In our project, each student was required to sign an agreement to work as an audiologist, speech-language pathologist, or teacher of the deaf in the Gaza Strip for three years after graduating. More than half of them didn't do so. The main reason was that the job market and the economy would not support the employment of all of our graduates. In this regard, the Minister of Health for the Palestinian Authority mentioned in his speech at the graduation ceremony that the Palestinian Authority hoped to hire all of our program graduates. Unfortunately it wasn't able to do so.

WHAT IS THE BENEFIT OF FORMING UNIVERSITY PARTNERSHIPS FOR INTERNATIONAL PROJECTS?

We found that a single university lacks sufficient resources to conduct a large project such as ours. By partnering and pooling resources, the project becomes feasible. This was the reason why Lamar University partnered with Marquette University for this project. Lamar University could not do it alone because at that time, Texas universities were not allowed to award external degrees unless the participating students obtained at least half of their university credits on a Texas campus. Furthermore, Lamar did not have sufficient faculty persons to teach all of the courses in Gaza. Marquette University, as a private institution, could award degrees to students who didn't attend classes on its campus. It could also provide faculty for some of the speech-language pathology courses that Lamar University couldn't. Marquette University, incidentally, couldn't have done the project alone because it didn't have faculty who were qualified to teach the deaf education courses.

HOW IMPORTANT IS IT TO PARTNER WITH A WELL RESPECTED INSTITUTION IN THE COUNTRY?

Doing so is likely to be essential for funding and other reasons. Both GOs and NGOs are more likely to fund a project like ours if it is administered by a well respected institution in the country that it's being conducted. This was certainly the case for our project. The USAID grant application was developed (with some assistance from one of us—RM) by the Society for the Care of the Handicapped in the Gaza Strip and the funding it yielded was awarded to the Society. Both Lamar University and Marquette University were sub-contractors and consequently, their contractual relationship was with the Society rather than with USAID.

There is at least one other reason why it's essential to partner with such an institution. Local governmental and non-governmental agencies are likely to be highly knowledgeable about how to get things done within the framework of the structure yielded by the country's history, culture, and politics. Consequently, it's more likely to be able to secure needed cooperation from both the government and the NGOs in the country than is a university (or group of universities) from outside of the country.

WHAT ARE SOME POTENTIAL FUNDING-RELATED PITFALLS AND HOW MIGHT THEY BE AVOIDED?

There are several. One is failing to budget for unforeseen expenses. While it's unlikely to be possible to anticipate all of them, the better you're able to do so, the more likely you are to have the funding needed to complete the project.

Differences in accounting practices can be a source of problems. It is likely, for instance, that a U.S.-based funding agent would expect U.S. accounting standards to be followed in a developing country even when such practices are quite novel to the people living in that country. Business practices that would be considered unethical and/or illegal in one country may be considered acceptable in an other and vice versa. A GO or NGO that makes a grant to an entity in a developing country and insists that the associated project be administered according to its rules is likely to have cause for complaint.

WHAT KINDS OF SUPPORT ARE STUDENTS LIKELY TO REQUEST FROM PARTICIPATING FACULTY AFTER GRADUATING?

Students in developing countries are likely to both need and request more support after graduating than ones in developed countries. In addition to the usual requests for recommendations for graduate school and jobs, they're likely to have a long-term need for advice from the faculty who taught professional courses, particularly if program graduates are the first persons in their community to practice their profession. This was the case for the graduates of our program. Some of our faculty continued to volunteer to consult with our graduates on professional issues by e-mail or fax for years after the end of the program.

Chapter 9

Do's and Don'ts for Planning Similar Projects

The main reason we wrote this book was to encourage the faculty and administration of at least a few universities in developed countries to explore the possibility of doing similar projects in developing nations. Such projects may train practitioners in fields other than rehabilitation and special education. And they may not be degree-granting programs. If this book facilitates at least one such project, we'll consider the hundreds of hours we've invested in authoring it as having been time well spent!

We've learned a great deal about what works and what doesn't from our involvement with this project as well as with other rehabilitation and special education practitioner-training programs in developing countries. We'll be sharing some of what we learned with you in this chapter. Hopefully, our doing so will make it unnecessary for you to have to "completely reinvent the wheel" if you decide to take on a project of this type.

The structure that we use in this chapter for organizing is do's and don'ts. The order in which the do's and don'ts are presented is not intended to communicate anything about their relative importance.

In order to maximize our ability to be helpful to persons planning similar projects, we distributed draft copies of this chapter to some of the others who taught in the program and asked for comments and additions. Consequently, the suggestions offered here are not all ours.

DO'S

Conduct the Program in Their Country Rather Than in Yours

Doing so can yield several benefits for students. First, it's apt to prepare them better to function professionally in their culture. Second, if practicum experience is a component of the program, the people in their country will benefit from it. And last, but certainly not least, it increases the likelihood that they will remain in their country after graduating—i.e., not contribute to its "brain drain."

Doing this can also benefit the participating faculty and institutions. It can provide a significant life-enhancing experience for faculty persons who participate (see Chapter 7). And it can enhance the image of participating institutions, particularly if the training program relates to healthcare or special education.

Select Intelligent, Motivated Students with Strong Leadership Skills Who Have the Ability to Work Independently

You're apt to have an easier time attracting such students for your program in a developing country than you are in your own. One reason is that, in a developing country, it's likely to be considered more prestigious to have a degree from a western than from a local university and few families in such countries can afford to send their children abroad for a degree. This means that you will have a larger pool from which to select the best and the brightest.

To nurture a profession, it is perhaps more necessary for the persons practicing it to have strong leadership skills and the ability to function independently in a developing country than would be the case in a developed one. It isn't enough for those who are the pioneers in a field to nurture it by maintaining the status quo. They have to go considerably beyond this if they are to be successful in getting it recognized and accepted in their society. And to do so they must have strong leadership skills. Furthermore, they're likely to have fewer peers with whom to consult (at least at first) and consequently, it's essential that they can work independently.

Maintain Standards That Are as Close to Those on Your Campus as Is Practical

You'll be doing your students no favor by "watering down" the training you provide. To function successfully as pioneers in their field, professionals in developing nations are at greater (certainly not less) need to be well trained than are those would-be professionals who are being trained on your home campus. Furthermore, if in a developing country young professionals have confidence in the quality of their training, they are more likely to work toward getting themselves and their new field respected and recognized.

Have Students Sign an Agreement to Work in Their Country in the Field in Which They're Majoring for at Least Three Years After Graduating

Such an agreement in a developing country is more likely to be enforceable "by conscience" or by societal pressure than by a court. A student from a developing country who signs such an agreement and fails to live up to it is probably at greater risk for losing respect in his or her community than is a student from a developed (capitalistic) country, particularly if the field for which the student was trained relates to healthcare or to special education.

Require Students to Pay Something for Their Education

People tend to value an education for which they pay something. The students in our program were each required to pay $1,000 toward the cost of tuition and books. With the average monthly salary at that time in the Gaza Strip being around $300, the $1,000 fee was a considerable sacrifice for the students and their families. Nevertheless, given that there were few viable alternatives in Gaza and knowing that, in the long run, the fee would prove to be a good investment, we felt justified in charging the fee.

If Possible, Have the Program Culminate in a Degree Rather Than a Certificate

There are a number of reasons for a degree being desirable, including the fact that degrees in developing countries tend to garner more respect for recipients than do certificates. Consequently, a person who has a university degree in a field is more likely to be successful at securing the cooperation and resources needed to nurture the field.

Consider Partnering with Another University

Only by partnering and pooling resources could Marquette and Lamar conduct this project. Neither institution could have done it alone. It's our impression that both institutions benefited sufficiently from partnering that they'd be willing to seriously consider a similar relationship again

Partner with an NGO in the Country that Is Both Well Respected by the Community and Influential with the Government

The success of our project was due in large part to the fact that we partnered with such an NGO (the Society for the Care of the Handicapped in the Gaza Strip). Doing so enabled us to secure funding for the Project from USAID and the support that we needed from the Palestinian Authority and from Israel.

If Possible, Make English the Language of Instruction

There are at least two reasons why making English the language of instruction is likely to be desirable. First, doing so should make it easier to secure faculty. The pool of potential faculty who speak English is likely to be larger than that for any other language. And second, doing so will provide the students with an essential tool for expanding their knowledge and keeping up-to-date. English is the language in which most professional books, journals, and Internet websites are written. Furthermore, it is the most useful language for communicating internationally by e-mail and it is an official language at most international conferences.

If English Is to Be the Language of Instruction and the National Language Isn't English, Provide Tutoring in English as a Second Language

If the field for which you're training students is to flourish in their community after they graduate, it is crucial that they be able to communicate well in English. They'll need this ability to expand their knowledge, keep up-to-date, and network internationally. Consequently, it could be as important for the students in your program to develop proficiency with English as it is for them to develop competence in certain of the skills needed for functioning in the field.

Anticipate a Considerably Higher Drop-out Rate Than You Would for a Similar Program on Your Campus

We began with more than twice as many students as we ended up with. This high a drop-out rate was neither desired nor anticipated by us. Most of it occurred during the first year.

Try to Anticipate Possible Contingencies When Planning the Budget

It is crucial that you give sufficient attention to developing a realistic budget. Seek all of the advice you can get. Economic uncertainty is too often the rule in developing countries and this makes it particularly challenging to estimate costs for multi-year projects. Understand too that the costs of goods and services can differ dramatically from country to country. If possible, stress these points with your funding agent(s) and request that periodic budget adjustments be possible.

Train Practitioners to Function Well in Their Community (Culture), Not Yours

What's necessary to have a successful practice in your students' community may differ in some significant ways from what's necessary in yours. For example, they'll probably have to be able to function with a lower level of funding and/or less technology than would comparable practitioners in your community. Then too, the services available in your community may not be available in your students' locale, or if they are offered, may not be of the same quality or offered at comparable prices.

Be Respectful of Differences Between Your Culture and Theirs

Never, never, never denigrate your students' culture! Thoughtless comments that cast dispersions on the students' homeland can do significant harm to your project. Remember, even well-meaning but slightly negative comments will be repeated outside of the classroom by your students and then further repeated again by family and friends. Do not be judgmental. Pre-employment training and in-service programs must make this point again and again. Few actions can damage an international training program more than making derogatory comments about culture, customs, history , economics, government, etc.

Orient Faculty about Cultural and Other Expectations for Them

It's crucial that this be done either before they leave their home campus or as soon as possible after they arrive. Some of the issues that should probably be dealt with are indicated in Appendix D.

Have a Formal Graduation Ceremony

Graduation is at least as much worth celebrating in a developing country as it is in a developed one. Consequently, it's important for the students, as well as their family and friends, that it be celebrated at a formal ceremony. If the students are receiving college degrees, both the students and faculty should wear caps and gowns *if wearing them is compatible with the students' culture.* We see a need to at least ask if, in the students' country, different customs and/or celebratory clothing would be acceptable or even preferable. You may even want to present an honorary degree to a worthy recipient in the country (see Appendix F). This person may be the commencement speaker.

Another potential benefit from having a formal graduation ceremony is increasing the level of awareness in the community of the availability of the service the students were trained to provide. A formal graduation ceremony being conducted by a foreign university in their community is likely to be given extensive coverage by local, national, and possibly even international, media.

Have the Name of the Field in Which a Student Majored Printed on His or Her Degree Certificate

Marquette University doesn't print students' majors on its Bachelor of Science degree certificates. This caused problems when some of our graduates applied for jobs in countries where western diplomas are not seen very often. It necessitated us having to write letters to both GOs and NGOs that we wouldn't have had to write otherwise. Consequently, we'd recommend including students' majors on their degree certificate if at all possible.

Have a Formal Plan in Place Before the Students Graduate to Provide Networking Opportunities for Them and Support for the Development of Their Field After They Graduate

This is something that we should have done. We should have realized that a great deal of networking and other support from us would be necessary for both our alumni in the Gaza Strip and the professions of speech-language pathology, audiology, and deaf education there to continue to develop. We've been providing it informally (without extramural funding) by e-mail and fax and plan to continue doing so long term.

DON'TS

Avoid Using Faculty Who Are Likely to Trigger "Ugly American" Type Stereotypes

Your faculty are likely to be the first persons from your country with whom most (perhaps all) of your students, the staff of the NGO with whom you're partnering, and some others in their community have interacted. Consequently, the stereotype that they have of persons from your country is likely to be affected significantly by their behavior. Lederer and Burdick (1958) alerted people to this reality more than forty years ago in their book, *The Ugly American..* Furthermore, they described behaviors that are likely to cause the stereotype to be negative.

The faculty who participate in your program will be informal ambassadors for your country, whether or not they choose to be so. Consequently, if at all possible, avoid using ones who are likely to reinforce an "ugly American" stereotype. Furthermore, you may want to recommend to participating faculty that they read *The Ugly American .*

Discourage Faculty from Becoming Involved Romantically with Students

Such dating is likely to be considered unacceptable by both the staff of the NGO with whom you're partnering and the students' families (see Appendix D).

Chapter 10
Research Implications: Questions Answered and Awaiting Answers

Most projects, including ours, have the potential to yield multiple benefits. Many of those that relate directly to our primary objective (i.e., training speech-language pathologists, audiologists, and deaf educators to manage the communicative disorders of persons residing in the Gaza Strip) were dealt with in previous chapters. Our focus in this chapter is on benefits that are research-related. Specifically, we present here a discussion of those research-related questions that seem to be answered, at least partially, by the lessons learned in this project. In addition we present a number of questions that we have not been able to answer definitively.

QUESTIONS ANSWERED

Can a Bachelor's Degree Program Be Successful in a Developing Country When the Partner Is a Local NGO Rather Than a Local University?

The fact that the local entity with whom we partnered was the Society for the Care of the Handicapped in the Gaza Strip rather than a university indicates that such a partnership can be viable for conducting a bachelor's degree program, particularly if the NGO has done so previously. The Society had been partnering with the University of Calgary for such programs for a number of years and, in fact, had one ongoing when ours began. The University of Calgary shared their classroom space and teaching equipment with us and, to a limited extent, we exchanged faculty.

Undoubtedly, our partnering with the Society went smoother because of the experience it had gained from partnering with the University of Calgary. However, the first training program on which the Society partnered with the University of Calgary was successful. This suggests that previous involvement with such partnering, while desirable, isn't essential.

Are Qualified Students in a Developing Country Likely to Be Attracted to Programs Like Ours?

Our experience in Gaza (as well as that of the University of Calgary there) suggests that large numbers of students are likely to be attracted to such programs, particularly if the university (or universities) with whom the local NGO is partnering are from a western country and the tuition is affordable. We had more than 200 applicants for our program. Degrees from western universities tend to be more highly respected in developing countries than those from local institutions of higher education.

Is it Feasible to Teach a Bachelor's Degree Program in a Developing Country in English When It Is Not the National Language?

Our experience suggests that it's feasible for English to be the language of instruction, particularly if you're willing to include classes in English as a Second Language in your program. And, as we've indicated previously, by helping your students to become more proficient with English, you're facilitating their ability to continue expanding their knowledge after they graduate.

Is It Possible to Find a GO or NGO to Fund Such a Program?

Our experience suggests that it should be possible to do so. However, if we were seeking funding in 2001, it's unlikely that we'd be able to get it from USAID. In 1994 or 1995, USAID apparently ceased giving grants to NGOs in the Palestinian territories. Beginning then, USAID gave whatever funding it had allocated for the Palestinians to the Palestinian Authority.

Can Private and State-Supported Universities Partner to Present Degree-Granting Programs in Developing Countries?

Our experience indicates that it 's possible for such a partnership to be successful as long as the administrations of both universities are willing to be flexible. One reason for the need for such flexibility in our program was that the Lamar University courses in deaf education for which students needed Marquette University credit were not offered by Marquette University.

Is It Possible to Secure Short-Term Faculty for Such a Program?

Both our experience and that of the University of Calgary indicate that it's possible to do so, even if where the program is conducted is perceived to be dangerous. The Gaza Strip was under military occupation and the Intifada was ongoing during most of the period when both we and the University of Calgary were recruiting short-term faculty to teach in Gaza. Furthermore, the U.S. State Department issued travel warnings for the Gaza Strip during most of the period that we were recruiting faculty to teach there.

Is It Feasible for Such a Program to Have a Liberal Arts Component?

Our experience suggests that it is not only possible, but desirable. It presumably facilitated our students' ability to think and reason rationally as well as their ability to think of themselves as educated professionals, rather than as trained technicians.

QUESTIONS AWAITING ANSWERS

It's highly unlikely that the data needed to answer any of the following questions will be generated in the near future through research specifically intended for this purpose. However, the data needed to provide at least a first approximation of an answer to some of them can probably be abstracted from reports of training programs (such as this one) that have been conducted in developing countries. Hopefully, the publication of this report will motivate others who have conducted such programs in developing countries to publish in-depth descriptions of them if they haven't already done so.

Is There Likely to Be Less of a "Brain Drain" If Students Are Trained on Site Rather Then in a Developed Country?

We assumed that there was likely to be less of a brain drain if we trained the students in the Gaza Strip rather than if we did so in the United States. This assumption was based on anecdotal reports of a huge brain drain when students from developing countries are trained in the U.S. For instance, we know that approximately 80 percent of U.S.-trained Chinese professionals remain in the U.S. after graduation. We're going to try to keep track of our graduates so that we'll be able to assess and report on the validity of our assumption at some later date.

What Is the Minimum Knowledge of English That It's Essential for Students to Have When They Begin the Program If English Is to Be the Language of Instruction?

It is our impression that, initially, most of our students would not have scored well on the Test of English as a Foreign Language (TOEFL) and, because of this, most would not have been admitted to a university in the United States. By the end of the four-year training program, however, given the ESL course work and the experience with English lectures and reading material, most of our students had mastered English to the point where they could succeed at graduate programs in the U.S. or in other English-speaking countries.

What Are the Options for Structuring English-as-a-Second-Language Instruction (Tutoring) for Such a Project?

We used daily classes and individual tutoring. The first few years of the program we had two full-time teachers of English as a second language. Later, we just had one. These ESL teachers established excellent relationships with the students and, consequently, the students didn't hesitate to ask for help.

What Kinds of Courses Can Be Taught Successfully During a Three or Four Week Period? What Kinds of Courses Can't Be Taught Successfully During Such a Period?

All 18 of the liberal arts core courses in our program and most of the professional ones were taught by short-term faculty during a relatively short period (3-4 weeks). There, of course, are courses that can't be taught so intensively. This is why we used both short- and long-term faculty.

What Is the Personality Profile of an Ideal Short- and Long-Term Instructor for Such a Program?

To answer this question it would be necessary to generate personality profiles for a number of faculty who were successful as short-term instructors and identify the characteristics that they share. It would be helpful when doing so to have personality profiles for at least a few short-term instructors who weren't successful.

What Approaches Are Viable for Recruiting Short- and Long-Term Faculty for Such a Program?

We used advertisements in national professional journals, group informational meetings for potential faculty at which at least one of the speakers was somebody who had already taught in Gaza, and individual "arm bending" meetings with potential faculty. There undoubtedly are other viable options for such recruiting.

What is the Personality Profile of an Ideal Student for Such a Program?

Our unintended high drop-out rate during the early stages of the Project is evidence of the need for developing such a profile. One item on it would undoubtedly be a high level of motivation to graduate from the program. If an applicant who had a high level motivation to do so was asked the following hypothetical question—"If you graduated from this program, how would your life be different?"—the answer he or she gave would indicate that the change anticipated would be both positive and huge.

What Approaches Are Viable for Recruiting Students for Such a Program?

We used advertising in local media and "word of mouth." There are undoubtedly other viable approaches.

What Attributes Should a Local NGO Possess to Make It an Ideal Candidate for a Partnership Like Ours?

Based on our experience, three such attributes would be having an excellent track record for attracting international funding, being both well respected in its community and influential with its government, and being willing to abide by the accounting practices and other regulations of the international GO or NGO that is funding the project.

What Are the Options for a University Seeking Another to Partner With?

Lamar University was able to locate a private university with which to partner for this project by "exploiting" the institutional affiliation of one of its adjunct faculty (FHS). While this strategy did yielded a positive result, there undoubtedly are more efficient and reliable ways for a university to locate such a partner. Perhaps advertising in a publication like the *Chronicle of Higher Education* would be one.

Appendices

Appendix A
Participants in the Project

One of the reasons we wrote this book was to provide a historical record of our training program. Consequently, it seems appropriate that we acknowledge each of those who participated in it as a student or faculty/staff member. The names of those who did so are listed below.

STUDENTS

Mahmood Abdel-Latif
Hussam Abu Ghali
Mysara Abu Hashem
Falastine Abu Jayyab
Mona Abu Moalek
Ahmad Abu Nada
Sami Abu Sultan
Kamel Ayad
Ayman Dawood
Akram Eid
Samy El-Alem
Yazdan El-Amawi
Mohammed El-Araeir
Mohammed El-Arouki
Ziak El-Askary
Mosa El-Khorti
Ne'mat El-Migati
Abed El-Monem Soboh
Abed El-Rahman El-Askary
Samar El-Ramly
Rae'da El-Wawi
Mohammed El-Zenjay
Mohammed Hamad
Mohammed Hamdan
Ahmad Hussein
Ramadan Hussein
Reem Nassrawi
Suliman Salah
Khetam Shakshak
Raja'a Sharaf
Nedal Shehada
Ashraf Yaghi
Naser Yousef

FACULTY/ STAFF

Aida Abu Ghazaleh
Hatem Abu Ghazaleh
Robert B. Ashmore
Kit Basquin
Steven C. Bourgeois
Kathleen Chinn
Kelly Dobbs McConnell
Renee Downs (Slette)
John Doyle
Sameer H. El-Isa
Robert Helmer
Julian Hills
Frank Hubbard
Tracy Kuberis
Frank Lazarus
Richard Logan
Lynn E. Miner
Robert Moulton
Thomas D. Oakland
Michael Pachuilo
Annette Powell
Muhammed (Sam) Randazo
John J. Schmitt
Franklin H. Silverman
Marshall Smith
Andrew Stuart
Andrew F. Tallon
Mary Beth Tallon
Michael Vater
Amal Zead
Michael Zeps

Appendix B
Curriculum

NOTE: In the interest of space, only abbreviated course descriptions are presented. Most of those for the foundation, speech-language pathology, audiology, and deaf education courses were abstracted from the USAID grant application for the Project. The descriptions for the 18 liberal arts core courses are from the *Marquette University 1995-1996 Undergraduate Bulletin.*

The students took all of the foundation, speech-language pathology, and liberal arts courses and some or all of the audiology and deaf education ones (depending on their choice of a second major). The professional courses in speech-language pathology and audiology were those required for certification by the American Speech-Language-Hearing Association. The deaf education courses were mostly those required for a deaf education major at Lamar University. And the courses that formed the liberal arts core were mostly ones that communicative disorders majors at Marquette University were required to take. The students were awarded fifteen semester hours of foreign language credit because they had acquired proficiency in English, in part, through courses in English as a Second Language.

SPEECH, HEARING, AND LANGUAGE FOUNDATION COURSES

Anatomy of the Speech Mechanism. Basic human anatomy and physiology related to normal respiration, phonation, resonance, and articulation. Students will develop an understanding of normal structure and function to enable them to recognize and appropriately deal with anomalies presented by the communicatively disordered. Students are required to acquaint themselves with the human skeleton, muscular system, nervous system, larynx, and skull.

Neuroanatomy and Neuropathology Relating to Communication Disorders. Course covers the nervous system, neurolinguistic correlates, causes of neurological problems and their impact on speech, language, and communication, and an overview of neurogenic speech and language disorders.

Speech Science and Phonology. Course covers the basic physics of sound, instrumentation in speech sciences, and acoustic phonetics. Students will be able to describe the basic parameters of sound, including frequency, intensity, the sound spectrum, and duration; identify instrumentation in acoustic phonetics; and describe the acoustic parameters of consonant and vowel production. Students will demonstrate a knowledge of phonetic and sociolinguistic factors affecting variations in production. Course covers instrumentation in audiology, speech-language pathology, and education of the hearing impaired. Students will demonstrate a knowledge of the principles of electricity and electronics. Students will understand transducers, audiometers, impedance bridges, tape recorders, instrumentation for physiologic assessment (evoked potentials, electronystagmography), signal generators and processors, and computers.

Sign Language. There are three courses that begin at the very basic fingerspelling level and progress through signing in Arabic, signing in Arabic Sign Language, and interpreting. Students will demonstrate an ability to converse and interpret in Arabic Sign Language. Students will demonstrate a knowledge of morphological and semantic considerations of Arabic Sign Language, the psycholinguistics of sign language, and education considerations (teaching Arabic as a second language, bilingual possibilities of Arabic Sign Language and Arabic).

Clinical Research Methodology. Course covers the information about the scientific method, statistics, and research methodology needed to both evaluate and do speech-language pathology, audiology, and deaf education research, with particular emphasis on outcome research. Students will demonstrate a knowledge of statistics and clinical research methodology adequate to both critically evaluate research in speech-language pathology, audiology, and deaf education journals and document the impacts of their clinical intervention and teaching on their clients and pupils.

SPEECH-LANGUAGE PATHOLOGY COURSES

Aphasia and Neurogenic Disorders. Course covers the nervous system, neurolinguistic correlates, causes of neurological problems and their impact on speech, language, and communication, and an overview of neurogenic speech and language disorders. Students will select appropriate assessment procedures and diagnostic features of neurogenic speech and language disorders; and select, explain and justify treatment procedures appropriate for different neurogenic speech and language disorders.

Voice Disorders. Course covers anatomy and physiology of the vocal mechanism, normal phonation, organic and functional voice disorders, diagnostic and screening procedures, alaryngeal speakers, voice characteristics of the aging, public school voice programs, and medical considerations. Students will identify and describe the anatomy and physiology of the respiratory and phonatory systems, and organic and functional causes of voice disorders. Students will select and describe appropriate techniques for training vocal skills in children and adults and for diagnosing voice problems.

Augmentative Communication. Course covers augmentative communication systems, historical perspectives, terminology, contemporary issues, population considerations, design considerations, computer technology, selection considerations, and methods of patient training. Students will discuss the decision process for adopting an augmentative communication system, be able to apply criteria for adopting augmentative communication given hypothetical cases, describe preliminary training strategies used with non-speaking children and adults, describe support services needed for severely handicapped clients, and discuss appropriate assessment procedures for the non-vocal client.

Children's Language Development and Disorders. Course covers an overview of language development and disorders in children, characteristics; causes and treatment of language disorders; assessment of cognitive, lexical, syntactic, and pragmatic skills; and language intervention strategies with preschool children, school children, and families. Students will discuss major characteristics of language development and disorders affecting semantics, morphology, syntax and pragmatics; be able to discuss the different purposes and types of assessment procedures used to identify language disorders in children; select appropriate language assessment procedures and tests relative to the child's age and domain; and select, explain and justify the use of intervention techniques used in training communication skills.

Articulation Disorders. Course covers phonological theory and acquisition, assessment of phonological disorders, and phonological intervention. Students will explain the critical aspects of current theories of phonological acquisition; describe the different stages of normal phonological acquisition; describe the characteristics of phonological disorders; explain the major causes of phonological disorders; score and interpret different assessment procedures for evaluating phonological disorders; plan and implement procedures to document generalization in therapy; discuss a hierarchy of phonological intervention and describe procedures appropriate at different stages of intervention; describe characteristics of motor speech disorders in children; and describe specialized approaches to training children with motor speech disorders.

Diagnostics and Counseling. Course covers the diagnostic process, the role of the speech mechanism evaluation in making a differential diagnosis, speech processes and disorders, and language and communication disorders. Students will demonstrate knowledge of diagnostic report writing; speech mechanism characteristics in making a differential diagnosis; advantages of norm vs criterion-referenced assessment procedures; appropriate procedures for language, fluency, articulation, voice and neurogenic communication disorders; and basic counseling principles relative to communication disorders.

Stuttering. Course covers theoretical perspectives and characteristics of fluency disorders, assessment and clinical management of fluency disorders. Students will differentiate between normal disfluency and stuttering; stuttering and cluttering; and stuttering and language formulation disorders. Students will describe characteristics of stuttering and stutterers; contrast a minimum of two different theoretical perspectives of stuttering; select appropriate assessment procedures for child and adult stutterers; outline counseling procedures to use with and describe at least one treatment approach for managing both fluency and stuttering in the chronic stutterer.

Cleft Palate and Other Craniofacial Disorders. Course concerns those craniofacial problems that impact on communication. Students develop an understanding of the anatomy and physiology of the craniofacial complex; normal and abnormal dental development; embryological development of the craniofacial complex;etiologies and incidence of cleft lip and palate; general surgical treatments of cleft lip and palate and the role of the speech-language pathologist in the rehabilitation team; dental/orthodontic treatments for cleft lip and palate; the various communication problems associated with cleft palate; and the various evaluative and therapy techniques for the communication problems associated with cleft palate.

Communication Disorders and Aging. Course covers demographics of the aging population; overview of the aging process; social realities of aging; physiology of aging; cognitive aspects of aging; effects of aging on auditory structures and processes; affects of aging on speech, language, and communication; communication problems of aging; and the diagnosis and treatment of speech, language and hearing disorders of the aging. Students will demonstrate knowledge of the normal aging process as it affects physiological processes, cognitive and social skills; and speech, language and hearing skills. Students will demonstrate knowledge of communicative disorders associated with the aging process, appropriate assessment procedures for evaluating auditory, speech, language, and auditory communicative skills for the aged population. Students will also demonstrate knowledge of appropriate intervention procedures for the geriatric population.

Clinical Practicum. Course repeated each semester. Supervised clinical experience with a variety of communication disorders.

AUDIOLOGY COURSES

Audiology. Course covers audiological evaluation, interpretation, referral, ramifications of hearing loss, and rehabilitation programs. Students will demonstrate knowledge of audiological terminology, standards, and equipment. Students will demonstrate an understanding of the format and integration of the auditory evaluation: speech tests, pure tone tests, and air conduction tests. Students will demonstrate an understanding of masking, impedance audiometry, and amplification.

Advanced Audiology. Course covers audiological evaluation, interpretation, referral, ramifications of hearing loss, and rehabilitation programs. Students will demonstrate knowledge of audiological terminology, standards, and equipment. Students will demonstrate an understanding of the format and integration of the auditory evaluation: speech tests, pure tone tests, and air conduction tests. Students will demonstrate an understanding of masking, impedance audiometry, and amplification.

Medical Audiology. Course covers medical aspects of auditory management. Students will show an understanding of the anatomy and physiology of the hearing mechanism (peripheral and central structures). Students will demonstrate a knowledge of anomalies, pathologies, diagnosis and treatment of external ear, middle ear, cochlea, and VIII nerve and central systems.

Bone Conduction and Masking. Course covers bone conduction theory, masking theory, impedance theory, and procedures and techniques associated with each. Students will demonstrate a knowledge of power/pressure dB notation and bandwidth development; masking theory, intensity, frequency and spectrum; modes and processes of bone conduction signal stimulation; procedures and techniques of clinical masking; calibration of bone conduction, masking, and impedance; theory of impedance test battery; and clinical applications of impedance batteries.

Special Audiometric Tests. Course covers the diagnosis of site of lesion and differential diagnosis. Students will demonstrate a knowledge of test battery development and test result integration. Students will show an understanding of the differential diagnosis process (peripheral structures vs. cochlear, and cochlear vs. retrocochlear). Students will demonstrate a knowledge of nonorganic hearing loss, central auditory testing, and test interpretation.

Electrophysiology. Course covers evoked potential audiometry and electronystagmography. Students will demonstrate a knowledge of neuroanatomy and the central auditory pathways; neurophysiology and resting potentials, graded potentials, and action potentials. Students will show an understanding of evoked potentials in auditory brainstem response, and middle latency response. Students will also show an understanding of electronystagmography and immitance testing.

Instrumentation. Course covers instrumentation in audiology, speech-language pathology, and education of the hearing impaired. Students will demonstrate a knowledge of the principles of electricity and electronics. Students will understand transducers, audiometers, impedance bridges, tape recorders, instrumentation for physiologic assessment (evoked potentials, electronystagmography), signal generators and processors, and computers.

Advanced Hearing Aids. Course covers the history of hearing aids; classification of hearing aids; components of hearing aids; special purpose hearing aids; standards; earmolds; hearing aid measurements; speech audiometry; hearing aid selection; hearing aid evaluation in adults, children, and special populations; hearing aid counseling; and dispensing hearing aids in private practice and clinical settings. Students will conduct hearing aid measurements of stock aids, make and modify earmold impressions, conduct hearing aid interviews, and interview hearing aid dispensers. Students will show a knowledge of the history of hearing aids, the components of hearing aids, national standards, ethical considerations of dispensing hearing aids, hearing aid evaluations, and laws affecting the dispensing of hearing aids.

Pediatric Audiology. Course covers auditory problems of children. Students will demonstrate a knowledge of the embryology of the auditory system, development of auditory behavior in the young child, disorders of hearing and syndromes in children, auditory evaluation of children, impedance audiometry, and auditory rehabilitation in the young population.

Advanced Auditory Rehabilitation. Course covers educational audiology, classroom acoustics, compensatory electroacoustic processing of speech, speech perception and sensorineural hearing loss, and auditory training procedures. Students will demonstrate a knowledge of education management for the hearing-impaired child, counseling parents of hearing handicapped children, laws and codes associated with classroom acoustics for the hearing impaired, group amplification systems and auditory training devices/techniques, the role of the audiologist in the educational setting, the adventitiously deafened, and the team approach to auditory intervention.

Clinical Practicum. Course repeated each semester. Supervised clinical experience with a variety of communication disorders.

DEAF EDUCATION COURSES

Speech Development in the Hearing Impaired. Course covers speech perception and development in the hearing impaired. Students demonstrate a knowledge of the history of teaching speech to the hearing impaired, current diagnostic and treatment procedures, common speech problems of the deaf and hearing impaired, speech assessment, and classroom intervention techniques.

Language and Deafness. Course covers language development and intervention with the hearing handicapped. Students demonstrate an understanding of the impact of hearing loss on language development, connections between language and reading, bilingual approaches to language development for the hearing impaired, assessment of language in the hearing impaired, and language curriculums for the hearing impaired.

Pedagogy and Deafness. Course covers legal considerations in educating the hearing impaired, parent and infant training programs, educational support systems, and classroom management considerations for the teacher of the deaf. Students will understand the processes of referral, assessment, eligibility, and placement of handicapped children. Students will show an understanding of placement considerations for the hearing impaired: residential, day school, self-contained, and mainstreamed classes. Students will understand how related services (speech therapy, transportation, medical, diagnostics, counseling, etc.) affect deaf education. Students will identify the roles played by support personnel in deaf education (aides, principal, supervisor, directors of special education, etc.). Students will understand classroom management in deaf education (scheduling, discipline, parent interaction, documentation).

Methods of Teaching Language to the Deaf. Course covers normal language development in hearing children; language development patterns and problems in deaf children; language intervention strategies; methods of utilizing the family and community in language development for the deaf; and current theories of the impact on communication systems and language development in deaf children.

Psychology of Deafness. Course covers the characteristics of the deaf community and causes of deafness, communication and language systems, the psychology of deafness, evaluation and teaching, and research and theory of cognitive development in the hearing impaired. Students will demonstrate an understanding of the deaf community, genetics and genetic counseling, Arabic Sign Language, psychodynamics surrounding diagnosis of deafness, impact of hearing loss on family structure, behavioral patterns associated with hearing loss, psychological evaluation of the hearing impaired, and research and theory relative to deafness.

Multihandicapped Deaf. Course covers prevalence, demographics, etiologies of deaf individuals with other educationally significant disabilities: mental retardation, deaf/blindness, learning disabilities, emotional disturbance, and motor/ orthopedic handicaps. Psychological evaluation, educational programming, curriculum, teaching methods and materials are also discussed. Students are able to describe the prevalence and demographics of the deaf multihandicapped population; the various disabilities which can accompany deafness and how these combinations affect behavior, education and rehabilitation; review curriculum and materials used with deaf MH populations; the unique social, psychological and linguistic needs of this population; the organizations which serve deaf MH individuals and their families; the legislation which affects this population; and considerations for evaluating the deaf MH population.

Reading and Language for the Deaf. Course covers the reading habits of deaf adults, reading achievement levels in the deaf population, reading theory applied to the deaf, reading acquisition for the hearing impaired, diagnostic and teaching techniques, the relationship between reading and writing, and reading materials used with the deaf. Students will understand how reading is acquired by the hearing impaired; how it is assessed with this population; how reading comprehension can be taught to the hearing impaired; how to set up a literacy environment in the classroom for the deaf; the relationship between learning to read and to write; locate reading materials for deaf children; and how to teach functional reading skills to the deaf.

Methods of Teaching Reading to the Deaf. Course covers the reading habits of deaf adults, reading achievement levels in the deaf population, reading theory applied to the deaf, reading acquisition for the hearing impaired, diagnostic and teaching techniques, the relationship between reading and writing, and reading materials used with the deaf. Students will understand how reading is acquired by the hearing impaired; how it is assessed with this population; how reading comprehension can be taught to the hearing impaired; how to set up a literacy environment in the classroom for the deaf; the relationship between learning to read and to write; locate reading materials for deaf children; and how to teach functional reading skills to the deaf.

Instructional Methods for Teaching Math, Social Studies, Science, Preschool, etc. to the Deaf. Course covers legal considerations in educating the hearing impaired, parent and infant training programs, educational support systems, and classroom management considerations for the teacher of the deaf. Students will show an understanding of placement considerations for the hearing impaired: residential, day school, self-contained, and mainstreamed classes. Students will understand how related services (speech therapy, transportation, medical, diagnostics, counseling, etc.) affect deaf education. Students will identify the roles played by support personnel in deaf education (aides, principal, supervisor, directors of special education, etc.). Students will understand classroom management in deaf education (scheduling, discipline, parent interaction, documentation).

Classroom Management. Course covers classroom management techniques specific to the deaf. Topics covered include acoustical considerations, manual communication in instructional settings, learning environments which best meet the needs of deaf children, the impact of hearing loss on learning styles, and behavior management techniques which have proven to work with deaf children.

Clinical Practicum. Supervised practical experience in teaching deaf in individual and group settings. This course is repeated each semester.

LIBERAL ARTS CORE COURSES

Introduction to Communication. A survey of communication principles and processes as they relate to interpersonal communication, small group communication, culture and communication, persuasion, communication in organizations, and mediated communication.

Expository Writing 1. An introduction to the basic principles of rhetoric and composition. Investigation of and practice in the methods of expository writing.

Expository Writing 2. A further introduction to the principles of rhetoric and composition. Investigation of and practice in the uses of written language in argument, persuasion, and critical analysis.

Survey of English Literature. An introductory survey to the British literary tradition, from the beginning to the latter part of the 18th century. Readings drawn from authors such as Chaucer, Shakespeare, Milton, Pope, Swift, Fielding, and Johnson.

Survey of American Literature. An introductory survey of American literary traditions, from the beginnings to the Civil War. Readings drawn from authors such as Bradstreet, Franklin, Wheatley, Emerson, Poe, Douglass, Hawthorne, Stowe, Melville, and Whitman.

History of Western Art. Historical survey of painting, sculpture, architecture, and the minor arts representative of the main contributions of Western civilization. Illustrated lectures and discussions.

Growth of Western Civilization 1. An interpretation of the evolution of Western society beginning with the ancient Near Eastern experience to 1715.

Growth of Western Civilization 2. An interpretation of the evolution of Western society from 1715 to the present.

Principles of Sociology. An introductory survey of the discipline including social structures, social institutions, social differentiation and stratification, social power, the processes of human interactions, and methods of sociological investigation.

General Psychology. Introduction to scientific psychology: biological bases of behavior; perception; principles of learning; intelligence and personality testing; current theories of personality; conflict; adjustment and mental health; interpersonal relations; social processes; applications of psychological principles to human affairs.

The Nature of Mathematics. Concepts of mathematics for liberal arts students. Emphasis on understanding and appreciating concepts rather than developing computational skills.

Introduction to Theology. An introduction to theology through questions and themes selected from the Bible, Christian tradition, and the thought of contemporary theologians.

Religion and Culture. Theological analysis of culture and the empirical study of religion. Role of religion in premodern cultures, cultural integration and secularization, cultural conflict and pluralism, Religious reflection and commitment in a changing cultural context.

Islam. Major trends of Islamic religious thought, practice, and worship. Readings from the Qur'an and other Islamic writings. Current issues and developments.

Logic. The goal of the course is to provide the student with an understanding of correct reasoning as it is employed in ordinary discourse. To this end, the course will study topics such as: terms and propositions, definitions, opposition, induction and deduction, reasoning and argumentation, fallacies in argument.

Philosophy of Human Nature. Investigation into the meaning of rational life. The course deals with the following four problem areas: human choice, human cognition, the affective, social, and spiritual dimensions of the human person, and the unity of the human being.

Theory of Ethics. An investigation into the moral dimension of human life. Among the topics considered are the norms of morality and the general process of moral decision making.

Oriental Philosophies. The major systems of philosophy of India and China including early Vedic and Upanishadic systems, Buddhism, Brahmanism, Hinduism, Confucianism, Taoism, and Zen. Emphasis on the key ideas of Eastern philosophy.

Appendix C

Notes on Teaching in Gaza—1995

One of the short-term faculty in the Program was Dr. Michael J. Zeps, S.J., an Associate Professor of History at Marquette University. During his first stay in Gaza, Dr. Zeps kept a diary (that he didn't intend to publish) in which he described his participation in the Program both candidly and graphically. Many of the experiences, reactions, and evaluations that he recorded in it were shared by us and likely also other participating faculty. Dr. Frank Hubbard, who is mentioned in the diary, is Associate Professor of English and Assistant Dean of the Graduate College at Marquette University . He was also a short-term teacher in the Program. We very much appreciate Dr. Zeps' willingness to allow us to reprint excerpts from his diary here.

****

May 16, 1995

Before I left for Gaza several people told me I ought to keep a diary of my experiences. I have been here for four days now and cannot promise to keep up on a diary, but I will record a few observations from time to time.

We left Milwaukee under adverse circumstances that were entirely avoidable. All the same, it was scarcely our fault. We never expected that rewriting a ticket could possibly take 45 minutes, but it did. The ticket agent...began sweating as the time grew shorter and the two of us stood there while the slips of paper piled up in front of him. He had to call somewhere to get directions on how to rewrite the ticket, had to refund money for traveling tourist rather than business class as the original tickets stipulated, had to apply that money to the cost of excess baggage in my case or charge extra money for excess weight in Frank

Hubbard's case, process the bills (we paid by credit card and so *more* slips of paper), get passports squared away, and negotiate with nervous baggage handlers as the time grew shorter and shorter. As we were boarding there was a last minute glitch; Frank Hubbard had locked his suitcases and they had to search them because of the destination. Upshot was that as we took off I looked out the window and saw our seven bags and boxes sitting on a cart. Inauspicious beginning. More to come.

The flight was uneventful. Connections in St. Louis were quick, which was probably the reason for the haste in Milwaukee. Connections in Paris-Charles de Gaulle were also expeditious which meant that there was no hope whatsoever that our bags would arrive with us. In Tel Aviv there were messages waiting for us to go to the TWA baggage counter. More paper work as we registered and described the lost bags. Luckily our ride to Gaza was still waiting patiently for us when we got through customs. Ah, but the weather was nice and has stayed perfect for us so far.....

Home is a fine new apartment that is very comfortable. The building is new enough that the stucco has not yet been applied to the concrete block exterior although it is old enough that the window in my room needed repair. Someone said it is a year old, but I would say it is more like four or five years old. The apartment is on the third floor, not a bad climb even for an oldster, has three roomy bedrooms, a living room, and one and a half baths. The kitchen is well appointed with a refrigerator, stove, and microwave. One of the bedrooms is our study with a Universal 486 computer and a fine printer that is better than anything I have in the States. The furniture, I understand, is all made at a furniture factory that employs the handicapped. It is sturdy and simple and the bed is comfortable, if not quite long enough for my frame. The overhead fans in all the rooms have not been needed yet because the weather is so perfect.

Things change from day to day around here. Today, for example, I got three different schedules within one hour and one of the staff was agitating for a fourth when I began to rebel. We get up around 6:30, have breakfast delivered around 7:15, get picked up by a driver around 7:45, and arrive at the college at 7:55. We start at 8:00, but the Palestinians have their version of the akademische Viertelstunde which gives me time to have things Xeroxed for distribution....

What we do is teach 33 students, all of whom are in the final year of a program in speech pathology and audiology. They are finally getting some liberal arts courses and the response is somewhat like dumping freshman courses on senior engineering students. They are busy with many things, and their schedules are so packed with practica, labs, and the like that they have little time to sit back and read. Of course English is their second language so reading is much slower. I had a choice of giving them a simplified textbook expecting them to read it all and giving them a solid text that they could keep and refer to later on even if they could not read it all now. I choose the latter....There are 21 chapters and we have 21 days, which works out neatly to one chapter a day. Compared with one chapter a week at MU that is a tall order for any student even if the text were simple and the native language English. So I flatter them even as I challenge them to the limit. I have been known as a tough teacher so why change now. They complain but they do all right. Had my first quiz today and the results were just about what I expected. Scores ranged from 15 to 4 on a 15 point quiz. That is just about the range I could expect from MU students. Nobody flunks, but the 4 is a D.

Teaching is vastly different, exhausting and delightful. These are really fine students. They have maintained their joy of life amid terrible adversity. Some of them have been in prison for agitation during the Intifada, and only one that I can determine has ever stepped foot beyond this strip of land only five miles wide and twenty-five miles long. They are totally engaged in the process of learning. Class is chaotic to a degree I have not seen since I taught remedial first, second, and third grade all together in one classroom during the summer of 1965, but these are young adults who know what they are about. There are two other teachers who are a great help to me, Sam who teaches English as a second Language (ESL) and Shelly who tutors them outside of class. That enables me to use the entire vocabulary of the English language as I do in a regular class at MU. I am more comfortable using words that express the nuances I see and then they explain the subtleties involved. It is a good system. Sam hit upon it. Sam and Shelly sit in on class and take notes, far better notes than the students, but they are struggling with English the whole time, not to mention my writing on the board.

That was the first minor confrontation we had. It happened the first hour of the first day. They wanted me to print on the board. But you can't write as much then. And I told them it is all right when you are explaining a word but not all right when you are putting whole thoughts on a board. Furthermore, they themselves have not been using cursive. So I bawled them out, extolled the virtue of cursive and said that second graders begin learning it. Anyway, they still have trouble with my writing on the board, but they are getting better. Who knows, maybe they will discover the benefits of writing, not printing, for themselves....But to be fair, there was a time, happily past, when American college students printed. I was appalled and bawled them out more acrimoniously than these students. What were they taught in grade school? Those same students did not know an adjective from a noun. These students do, so in the grammar department they are ahead of those dunderheads from the 70's and early 80's.

So much has happened in four days that I forget only a little time has passed. Our schedule for eating has changed after two days. No surprise there, of course. Two other teachers from the States have arrived. They teach speech pathology and audiology classes in the afternoon. We have lunch together at the Sun Center (not to be confused with the college) where the handicapped kids go to school....Before we ate there they delivered lunch to us here at the apartment. That was kind of neat, to come home to a cool, breezy sunny apartment and have a wonderful hot dish of chicken, potatoes, peas, and zucchini waiting for you on the table.

I will continue this later. Arab music is something else. I have been analyzing the music of the calls to prayer five times a day. Interesting! But more later.

May 21, 1995

Here it is, already five days later and I'm just getting back to writing....Things are settling down to an uproar at school. The schedule has been straightened out. Sunday through Wednesday we have one schedule and Thursday and Saturday another. In the former we are finished at 1:30 and then go to the Center for lunch. Thursday and Saturday we finish at 12:30 and then go to lunch, Thursday at home and Saturday at the Center. On Thursdays the staff gets off early so they deliver our meal to our apartment and we find it there when we get home.

The muzzein just got going again. They blast those calls to prayer on loudspeakers all over the city. I sleep through the early morning ones, as I do the first rooster calls. Funny, but a lot of things remind me of growing up in Milwaukee. They have chicken coops and pigeon coops here just like some of our neighbors did on 30th street. There are street vendors driving by hawking watermelons and other vegetables. But the calls to prayer are something new. A Bedouin woman browsing her herd of goats through the middle of town is something new, too. The goats eat just about anything, around here garbage and whatever....

Anyway, back to school. The classes are a constant buzz of noise but the students are totally engaged in what you are saying. They are always asking questions, some infuriating like asking me to explain something I just finished explaining, some quite profound like the one about the need for law codes like Justinian's if you have a religious consensus. They are very interested in religion and spirituality....The quizzes have improved. Maybe they are too easy. I doubt they are studying harder. There simply is not enough time for them to do everything in their schedules. But they are getting educated. They have a tough year ahead of them with the course of study we have planned for them. Condensing this course into three weeks has me chasing around like mad. But discipline in class is a problem. They get up and move around and talk constantly. A lizard got killed in class this morning. Somebody pulled a shade and it dropped on the floor. Poor thing. I felt sorry for it.

They certainly can have fun. Yesterday we had a going away party for Kathy at the beach. It was held at a new restaurant called El Saeed, with a glottal stop in the middle of course. They had a long table set up with place settings and a boom box. Nothing more was needed. They danced up a storm, laughed, joked, talked, and drank Royal Crown cola....

We are physically safe but it is still scary to see so many AK-47's around. Dr. Hatem, the guy in charge and something of a politician, stepped out of his office at the Center with us and called loudly for somebody. Two guys were there in an instant, his driver and a bodyguard with an AK-47 slung over his shoulder. They eyed us sharply. Yasir Arafat's compound is near the restaurant we were at yesterday and there are soldiers everywhere toting automatic weapons. Sandbagged emplacements with automatic weapons clearly visible are all around the place. Today there was a jeep ahead of us with an officer and three soldiers carrying M-16's that stopped and unloaded in front of an apartment building. The presence of fully armed troops in the middle of an urban setting is disconcerting. I'm not used to that. Checkpoint Erez is another unpleasant place. We've been through it four times so far. Maybe we will get to Jerusalem where there are even more soldiers. I would like to see the Dome of the Rock as well as the sacred Christian sites, but we may not get there. We'll see. The students also appreciated me saying that the Dome of the Rock, on the site of the Jewish Temple, is considered such an architectural masterpiece in the West that public opinion would be very much against doing any damage to it. They may have wondered why it has not been blown up already. That may help to explain it. To be this close to the Holy Land and not be able to see the places would be sad, but we are really busy with little free time. Anyway, I have to work on a test. A fifty minute test is not easy to work up and I have two to make up by day after tomorrow.

Well, I gave a test on Tuesday and it is Thursday May 25, 1995 now. I corrected the matching quickly but was just too tired to do the essays for the next day. Gave they back today and the results were mixed. The B class did pretty well and the A class not so well, but the tests were different and perhaps the A class had the tougher test. Then again...

On Tuesday, second hour, we had an Israeli from Tel Aviv University come and speak to all of the students about deaf education in Israel. It was something of a presentation of job opportunities for graduates of programs such as ours. There was a sharp exchange as the B class came back into the room. Sulieman seemed to be feeling strongly about something. He was jailed for two years during the Intifada, I hear. He seemed to be in a minority, though. Somebody else told Frank [Hubbard] he was not getting educated to make a contribution to Israel and I must confess a similar thought crossed my mind. But a job is a job when you are in need. It's not all black and white.

We went to a rug producing place on Monday and I ordered two specially made rugs for Lake Five. I was having trouble finding 3 foot by 8 foot runners for the big room. Could have had them custom made for $250 apiece in the States but I ordered two of that length here for a total of $55. Not as high quality, but at one fifth the price. Tried to arrange picking them up today but failed. They will have to wait until Saturday. I am at the mercy of the Center for providing transportation since I am completely in the dark as to where we were. The total lack of street signs of any sort doesn't help at all. The factory was interesting. All hand woven, the rugs were being produced by guys at looms right there. Frank bought two.

But the real reason why I wanted to write today—and I better do it quick because I'm fading—is to record impressions of our trip to Jabaliya Camp yesterday with Abed.... He invited us to the camp where there was a large Israeli military camp and where a lot of disturbances occurred during the Intifada. He and Ziad live there with their families and the family of another brother. First we took a taxi to Palestine Square where we walked in search of another taxi to take us north to Jabaliya City. The difference between Camp and City is not immediately apparent to me unless Camp refers to Jabaliya as a dumping ground for

Palestinians expelled from Israel after 1948 and City refers to the same one and one-half square kilometers now that it is covered with cinder block houses. Anyway, we got this big Mercedes taxi whose driver said to Abed that the was going that direction because he was going home for lunch. Maybe yes, maybe no. One old man came along. We accelerated to above 50 mph in the short straight-aways and wound our way tortuously through back alleys when we hit a construction site that was—illegally according to Abed—blocking the road. Then we inexplicably stopped and picked up three ladies, two of them of advanced years. The taxi had two back seats so three of us crammed into the back seat with the three ladies ahead of us. We careened off in another direction, quite different from the one that would take us to our destination according to Abed, and eventually let the ladies out. They did not pay anything. I was thinking that the taxi driver was a charitable soul until we got to the point where Abed suggested we start walking to get the flavor of the camp. When we got out the driver kicked the old man out along with us. We had already paid and that included the old man. Abed said that the driver simply did not want to take the old man any farther. So much for the charitable driver. Everything is different around here.

Abed first took us to a cesspool where the Israelis had herded several hundred Palestinians during the Intifada, pushed them down into a depression filled with sewage and started firing into them. Abed was one of them but "survived," as he said. He mentioned a couple of people he knew, one with 16 wounds who survived and one with just one who died. He said he had both legs broken by the Israelis during the Intifada. Afterwards I began to think of just how he survived and concluded it might well have been by ducking under the water of the cesspool. It was absolutely foul. The pictures I took will not communicate what the place was like. We then walked past schools and through densely packed alleys where the houses all had pictures on them of members of the family killed during the Intifada. We stopped for some Arab sweets at what passes for a sidewalk cafe and sat outside, a real innovation according to Abed. Some boys baited us by saying, "Shalom," perhaps thinking we were Israeli. We passed the school where Abed spent 6 years and the school where his father taught for 38 years (even Abed was amazed by this). Schools are segregated here and they were just getting out. We went through a crowd of secondary school girls, all in something approaching a uniform although the shawl was the only exactly uniform part of their dress and finally we found ourselves going the same direction as four mouthy little girls of about 8 or 9 who wanted their pictures taken and kept jabbering so much that they gave Abed a headache. "Just like old women," he said. Finally he asked the rudest one of them what her name was. She told him it was Ruoida whereupon he immediately told her he was going to tell her father. She didn't believe that Abed knew her father and asked him what her father did for a living. Abed was shrewd enough to duck that one so when we turned off the little girl came running up behind us and denied her name was Ruoida. She said it was Nema. But he had her scared so we got some measure of revenge. I'll bet the little pack of harpies was making uncomplimentary remarks about the two camera-toting foreigners, But Abed was too polite to tell us what they were saying.

We went through banks of houses separated by only four or five feet, nearly hit out heads on open shutters sticking halfway into the passage, and finally came to Abed and Ziad's house. So many things remind me of California around here and although Jabaliya City is incredibly dirty and crowded, once we were inside the house it was as though we were sitting in a quiet California Courtyard with citrus trees and neat flower beds. They have three families in the house but it is really a nice place. Ziad has an office with a computer in it, while eight kids and one adult were playing a game of ski jump on another computer. We had a glass of orange soda in Ziad's office then went outside and sat on the walk between the gardens and had first a wonderful mint tea with wafers then plums and peaches. I asked about the infrastructure and the vast amount of building that is going on everywhere in Gaza and got very informed answers. Since it was getting on to 7:00 P.M. and I had not corrected the essays yet I said we should be going. They gave us a quick tour of the house. We met Ziad's and Abed's wives, saw the beautiful baby Yousef, met a bunch of the kids and saw how crowded everybody is. Abed, who has a couple of kids from his brother's marriage when he married his widow, does not want more kids but Ziad said "Why not?" when asked if he wanted more. Then they drove us home. Ziad had clinic earlier or he could have driven us to Jabalya but then we would have missed the taxi ride out there. I am thinking now that maybe we should have invited them up but then I never would have gotten finished with the tests.

The students are making progress and follow my lectures with much more interest than American students. They are always stopping me and asking for clarification and when I make good points I have their rapt attention. Needless to say there are few good points because the periods of rapt attention are precious few. Mostly there is a low buzz that I have to shout over. And they always shout "Doctor," when my back is turned as I write on the board, often to ask me about the point I intended to make with the next breath. You'd think they would learn to hold their questions until the end. But who can fault such engagement with the material? Sometimes they repeat out loud what I am writing on the board. Then there are the questions about what I just finished explaining; at that point it gets maddening....

Well, we went to Jerusalem and Bethlehem yesterday....The students wanted to hear all about it today. I indulged the A class but kept the B class to their work. They ask so many questions in the course of class that I would never get any material covered if I went off on tangents. They tried to get me off on a tangent when I mentioned the Babylonian Captivity of the Jews! And Nebuchadnezzar!! Curious reactions around here. They seen thrilled that somebody they knew actually got out of Gaza to a place they considered their own. And Arabs over there are a lot different. These here have suffered a lot more and are more isolated. They seem more open and friendly, less grasping, and commercial than the people in Jerusalem. But we were in tourist country where everybody is greedy....

It is now June 2. Yesterday was their version of April Fools but they did not try anything on me. Just told me about it. The trip to some historical sites in Gaza seems to be on for tomorrow, but you never know around here. Sam is so hesitant about everything that it has been agony getting him to line up transportation. He wanted to know where we would be every minute because he was afraid of this and afraid of that. He circles around things and has a lot of trouble getting to the heart of the matter. A real nurturer, not a hard boiled administrator whose chief goal is to get something done. Anyway, Frank and I went to see some sites with Dr. Samy the day before yesterday. Dr. Samy (that's his title and first name) went to Princeton, got his Ph.D. from Syracuse in civil engineering, runs Gaza College, the local college prep school from which at least one of our students, Nedal, is involved in politics to the extent of going to Jerusalem several times a week, and is interested in history. Besides that he speaks perfect English. In other words, he is a great role model for our students. He did not have to come back to Gaza while many of our students want to get out of here desperately. Now I know from experience what a "brain drain" can be like. None of the students seem to have any hope for Gaza despite all the building and so forth. We went to some sites protected not only by signs saying, "Archeological site, no entrance" but by guards armed with AK-47's as well. Seems the Israelis took out as much as they could find including a completely intact Byzantine church covered by wind blown sand. The sites are interesting. Then we went to an old church—very interesting. Afterwards we went to the home of one of the guys showing us around, had small, raw zucchinis, tea, soda and saw his private collection—one spectacular, completely intact jug, a few old and very beautiful pieces of glass, and a few coins....

Three days ago we went around with Mohammed El-A. and saw a mosque that dated from 1443 and the Mosque at the Palace of Helena which we had seen from a different perspective on our trip with Nasser. Went up to the site overlooking the city where there was also an ancient Christian ruin (not much there) and took some pictures. His brother has a car and was driving us around so we stopped at his house and sat in the garden filled with olive trees and other California-style vegetation and had soda, tea, and fruit. That seems to be the order of hospitality, soda first, then fruit or small, raw zucchini and then tea. The pattern has repeated itself now in three places, Abed's, Mohammed's and our seaside friend. You can sure get a lot of agricultural produce from this land, sandy and poor though it appears. The sun is always shining, it seems, and the fresh water comes from somewhere in enough quantity to keep things irrigated....

The last thing we did on the trip with Mohammed was visit the hospital where his brother works as a practical nurse in the neonatal unit. We went in and toured the unit. The guys on duty, all men, were not exactly thrilled to hear we were Americans but warmed up a bit when they find out we were not doctors. The unit has modern equipment, but is congested and probably (that's the saving word) far below acceptable western standards....People in the crowded waiting area outside thought we were doctors and one couple came up carrying a tiny child with some awful white patch on its skull as we were leaving the unit. After all, we had been dressed up in green hospital garb to see the tiny infants and they could see through the door. In the States we would probably have been denied any access whatever to the neonatal unit. Things are different here.

Speaking of kids, you have never seen so many kids in one spot in your life. There are thousands upon thousands of them everywhere. An ordinary cluster of kids will run to 15 or 20 when you begin actually to count them. Simply incredible. The older ones take care of the younger ones. Few mothers to be seen outside the houses, just kids. And we never saw a woman (except when we toured Abed's house) when we were visiting. Lots of men of all ages, all of them very friendly.

But that friendliness has its limits, especially when it comes to kids. We went shopping yesterday to Palestine Square and on the way home we passed a kid who yelled, "Shalom!" at us like the kids had done to bait us when we were with Abed in Jabaliya City. Then he shouted, "Shalom!" to a friend across the street and when we were some distance away a couple of stones landed at our feet from two different directions. So Frank's T-shirt that says "I got stoned in Gaza" can be worn in all honesty....

Well this is the last day I am here. It is Monday, June 5 and I have finished giving my test. I did not check it very well last night and there were two mistakes in the test for section B. In addition there was one item, Louis IX, that showed up on both pages of matching, which gave them an edge. With all the pressure I have been under getting these things finished it is not surprising in a way, but still I should have checked things more closely. Was just too tired. Said fond farewells to lots of the students. I got to like them very much in this short period of time. Maybe I'll be back for History 002 if nobody else can take it in August. Not that I can take it then, but if they put it off to next year at this time I could come. It would be great seeing these students again at the end of their Marquette career. Could even stay for graduation. Whew! But his was hectic. Frank and I worked our buns off teaching four hours a day six days a week and cramming courses into three weeks. But we pulled it off....

It has been a wonderful experience. Maybe I can come back. It will be great to see the place when it has been cleaned up and the streets have been paved. But it won't be the same. The students will be older, wiser and more serious. Isn't that sad! Why can't they stay young all the time? And why can't we stay young along with them? Well I'm trying anyway.

Appendix D

Welcome to Gaza Packet

Let us begin by thanking you for your interest in our project to train Palestinians in the field of Communicative Disorders. We are glad to report the Project's advancements: there is a thriving audiology clinic, a "college" of communication disorders, and a home intervention program now in progress.

As our contracted staff approach their time of departure for Gaza we receive many questions regarding what to bring, wear, etc... We hope to answer many of these questions here, but feel free to contact Dr. Bob Moulton...

WHAT TO PACK?

CLOTHES

This depends mostly on the time of year you will be visiting Gaza. In general the weather is mild and pleasant. Extremes of heat and cold are tempered by the nearby Mediterranean Sea.

WINTER: low 30's to mid 40's (F) with occasional cooler weather. Your main problem will be the rain; so be prepared for wet weather December through most of February. A very heavy coat may not be necessary, but an all-weather, lined coat would be ideal. Gloves, long underwear, and heavy socks will come in handy this time of year, even indoors.

SPRING: low 50's to 70's (F). In the spring of 1994, Gaza experienced a brief record-setting heat-wave when temperatures reached 100 for a few days and then we experienced a sand storm. That was an exception, however, and spring is usually very enjoyable. You will rarely find a need for a coat, but sweaters are nice. Being close to the Mediterranean Sea, humidity can clash with the dry/warm air and result in an occasional rain shower. Gaza sits on the beach. The water stays fairly warm and you can swim even in the spring. Swim suits? No problem for men, but local custom prohibits revealing swimsuits for women (girls do swim, but only "fully-clothed"). However, it is just a short drive to Israeli beaches where there are no restrictions as to swimming attire.

SUMMER: mid 70's to high 90's. Most places will not be air conditioned. Be prepared with light-weight clothes; preferably made of cotton. A great shirt for men is the Polo style shirt and Levi Docker style slacks. Men are allowed to wear anything: shorts, tank-tops, swimming bikinis, etc.. Women must always be more cautious about their clothing, particularly outside of SCH buildings. A woman should be primarily concerned with the neckline and a shirt should be worn outside the pants and extend considerably below the waistline. The people really don't care to see a woman's elbows, but it is just too hot to wear long sleeves. Sleeves cut right above the elbows are acceptable, but never wear a tank-top or sundress.

FALL: mid 60's to low 80's, with weather turning cooler in November. There might be occasional rain storms during this time, but the main time for rain is during winter. A light jacket might be needed towards the end of fall. Also, the humidity might still be relatively high during this time, producing some foggy mornings.

While teaching or consulting, the staff can wear sport-dress style clothing. A coat and tie is not expected. Dress jeans are acceptable. Also, bring comfortable shoes, you might do a lot of walking. When traveling in Israel, anything is acceptable for both genders.

PERSONAL/TOILET ITEMS

Such items as shampoo, conditioner, aftershave, soap, etc. are available in Gaza or the nearby town of Ashkelon, Israel. Ashkelon has a small mall with a drug store similar to a Walgreens or Eckerds. Feminine products can be purchased there. A good idea is to pack enough of the above to last 2-3 weeks and by then you should know your way around Gaza and how to use the taxi service into Israel. Sometimes rides with United Nations employees are available into Israel.

Electrical appliances are usually provided in SCH-controlled flats and apartments. These include: hair dryers, radios, washing machines, microwaves, electric tea pots, and computers. A battery-operated alarm clock is a great idea to bring due to the many power outages that occur in Gaza. If there is a particular type of music you are found of, bring cassettes. The radio stations carry mostly Arabic tunes.

SCH is currently working on the Communication Disorders library for the facility. You may be asked to be a courier in this effort; the books are normally purchased in the States and then brought to Gaza by contracted employees. The books should be packed in your luggage; you will be allowed three check on bags.

Upon your arrival in Tel-Aviv, go through the green line of Customs Declaration. This line is for "NO DECLARATIONS." The security at the airport might ask you a few questions, but prepare for an intensive security check upon your departure from Gaza. Most persons leaving Gaza through Tel-Aviv will spend an hour or more answering questions at security. Usually, the security personnel are college-age and very polite, but it is a hassle to keep answering the same questions over and over again. If you are asked by SCH to carry in books, teaching supplied, hearing aids, etc., and if you are asked, these are donations from the U.S.A. (not items for resale).

WHAT TO DO IN GAZA ?!

THE UNITED NATIONS REC HOUSE "THE BEACH CLUB"

The UN REC House is where you will meet internationals and have the most opportunity for socializing. By the way, REC does not stand for recreation, it means Rescue and Evacuation Center. It is very important to have your name and address placed on the evacuation list at the REC House. The UN soldiers are responsible for the list and getting you out of Gaza in case of an emergency. So when the REC House is not acting as a rescue and evacuation center, it is the social hang-out for most internationals. There is a bar, television room with satellite, and a dining room (the food is not bad, but a little expensive). There is a membership fee: $35 for six months, $60 for a year, and you must speak to the manager for shorter memberships. The Palestinians know the REC House as the "Beach Club," so if you take a taxi just say "Beach Club" and you should get there. It is on the beach, but it is not a private beach. All the rules still apply: anything goes for the men but women must be fully clothed while on the beach. There are sun decks at the club for sunbathing. Women are allowed to dress anyway they choose within the club. That is, except for nude sunbathing, unless you are really brave. Saunas are also available and cost $2 a session. By the way, everything you purchase must be purchased with coupons. The coupons are purchased at the front desk. Shekels (NIS) or US dollars may be used to purchase the coupons.

THE FRENCH CULTURAL CENTER

If you are interested in taking Arabic lessons, this is the place for you. They teach both Arabic and French. It is in the general area of the Beach Club, about a mile from the Club. The Center will often show movies, but they are usually in French. So if you want to brush up on your French, they welcome all internationals to movie night. Ask any of the secretaries at SCH for the telephone number of the Center if you are interested. Arabic lessons will run approximately $30-$40 (100-150 NIS) a month depending on the size of the class.

RESTAURANTS

There are several restaurants in Gaza that are pretty good. Most restaurants are on or near the beach. The Palm Beach is highly recommended and inexpensive. You may spend at the most $3 for a very filling meal. They serve the traditional k-bob and shawarma sandwiches. But they also have some American-style dishes: hamburgers/fries, fried chicken, fish, steak, etc... The Lido serves good seafood, although it is slightly expensive. The Salaam restaurant also serves seafood.

SHOPPING

If you are living at SCH, light shopping will be relatively easy for you. There is a produce stand, grocery store, and bakery within 1-2 blocks from you. Purchasing meat is another story; WARNING: BE CAUTIOUS. There is a saying among the internationals in Gaza: If it does not even attract flies, it must not be good! The best thing to do is to purchase meat in Ashkelon or ask the locals from whom they trust to buy their meat.

An interesting thing to do is to visit Omar Mohtarh Street. Along the street there are many shops and this is where all the locals do their shopping. This street will give you a good dose of the local culture. The shop owners are very nice and will always ask you to come into their store and look around. Warning: since you are a foreigner, they might want to overcharge you. If it sounds too expensive, it probably is. Be careful about bartering, some take offense if you try. It is better just to refuse and go to a different store. You probably can find the same item cheaper somewhere else.

WHAT TO DO OUTSIDE GAZA ?!

ASHKELON

Ashkelon is a small town in Israel, just north of the border. It is about a 30 minute drive. In Ashkelon, there are two shopping malls. They have: movies, restaurants, a large grocery store, drug store, and clothing stores. It's almost like a little piece of home. If you like to play tennis, there is a very nice tennis center. I think it is about $5 to $10 to reserve a court for the evening. Also, there is a nice beach area there with a board walk (well, it is made out of cement). Both men and women can swim there in their swim suits. You may also visit the national park and tour the ruins within the park.

JERUSALEM

Everybody should visit Jerusalem! It is a neat experience to see the Old City and visit all the sites. Once you're inside the Old City its very easy to find a tour guide; actually, they will find you. Just look like a tourist and they will approach you. But be sure to ask how much for the tour before you start because they will take you for all you're worth if you don't. There are many things to see and do in Jerusalem. A good thing to do before you leave the States is to pick up a guide book for Israel.

THE SEAS

Besides the Mediterranean, there is the Red Sea, the Dead Sea, and the Sea of Galilee. Each place is very different. These places allow for swimming, scuba diving, and snorkeling.

FINALLY:

For a variety of cultural, religious, and political reasons, SCH desires that interactions between international employees and the local Palestinians be characterized by both friendliness and professional distance. It is expected that internationals will be polite and respectful of the local people and their customs. Romances between internationals and Palestinians, particularly Palestinian students and SCH staff, are strongly discouraged. While it is appropriate to meet with groups of students before and after class and to participate in extracurricular group activities; meeting alone with a student, particularly one of the opposite sex, is greatly frowned upon. Be careful how you respond to invitations to visit and dine at Palestinian homes. Palestinians are renowned for their hospitality and you will receive requests for socializing. Just remember the SCH policy on maintaining a professional demeanor and understand that the financial condition of most of the students is such that entertaining guests could mean considerable family sacrifice. Of course, you are free to socialize with the many non-Palestinians associated with the U.N. and other international agencies.

Appendix E
Representative "Letter of Agreement" Between SCH and Faculty

Dr. Franklin H. Silverman and Dr. Hatem Abu-Ghazaleh, Chairman of the Society for the Care of the Handicapped in the Gaza Strip (SCH), concur with the following letter of agreement.

1) Dr. Franklin H. Silverman shall be employed by SCH to perrform teaching and speech-language pathology consultation duties in Gaza December 27, 1993 through January 22, 1994 and to perform other related duties as assigned. Dr. Silverman will coordinate his teaching with the SCH/Lamar University program which trains audiologists, speech pathologists, and teachers of the deaf. His duties will be performed primarily in the SCH lecture facility in Gaza. Dr. Silverman shall be supervised by Dr. Hatem Abu-Ghazaleh, Dr. Robert Moulton, and/or SCH administrators designated by Dr. Abu Ghazaleh.

2) The Society for the Care of the Handicapped in the Gaza Strip will pay Dr. Franklin H. Silverman US$4,000 for his professional duties for December 27, 1993 through January 22, 1994. In addition, SCH will provide Dr. Silverman with one round trip airfare from Milwaukee, Wisconsin to Tel Aviv, Israel. SCH will provide Dr. Silverman's meals and lodging during his stay in Gaza at a cost to him of US$1,000. Dr. Silverman will be expected to follow the six day work week which is traditional for Gaza.

3) Since the Gaza Strip is within Israeli Occupied Territory, Dr. Silverman should not be considered at fault should political/military actions and/or other local conditions preclude him from teaching or otherwise performing his duties. If, for instance, the U.S. government determines that U.S. citizens should leave the Gaza Strip, and should this occur before he completes his teaching duties, SCH will pay Dr. Silverman on a pro-rated basis for the time he has worked and provide him with airfare to his home in the continental U.S.. Also, should strikes, curfews, or other local factors prevent Dr. Silverman from performing his duties in Gaza, he will receive his salary while he remains in Gaza and employed by SCH, though he may be required to alter his work schedule to compensate for lost time.

Dr. Franklin H. Silverman	Dr. Hatem Abu-Ghazaleh Director, Society for the Care of the Handicapped in the Gaza Strip
Date	Date

Appendix F

Citation for Dr. Hatem Abu-Gahzaleh's Honorary Degree from Marquette University

Dr. Hatem Abu-Ghazaleh, surgeon, humanitarian, philanthropist, educator, and peacemaker, has truly been a person for others.

As Founder and Chairman of the Society for the Care of the Handicapped in the Gaza Strip, Dr. Hatem has provided more than 6000 children living there with high-quality educational, rehabilitational, vocational, and medical services. He has established schools and clinics, as well as sheltered workshops and other enterprises to provide care for children and employment for his countrymen. These activities have been funded by grants from a number of governments, including those of the United States, Canada, Australia, Saudi Arabia, and Japan, as well as by his own family's financial resources.

Many more children with disabilities will be receiving rehabilitation services through the partnerships he has forged with several Canadian and United States universities, including Marquette, to train Palestinian rehabilitation specialists in Gaza. Marquette University faculty have gone to Gaza and taught liberal arts and other courses to the first group of students to be educated as speech-language pathologists, audiologists, and teachers of the deaf. These students will be receiving Marquette University baccalaureate degrees at their graduation this summer in Gaza.

Furthermore, Dr. Hatem has worked for many years to break down the walls of mistrust between Israelis and Palestinians. His selfless devotion to the needs of children with disabilities has earned him the respect, friendship, and support of many Israelis, including government officials.

For these reasons, Reverend President, I hereby recommend Dr. Hatem Abu-Ghazaleh for the Marquette University degree of Doctor of Laws, *honoris causa.*

Appendix G
Participants' Anecdotes

A number of the Americans who participated in the Program kept diaries while in Gaza or wrote about some of their experiences after returning to the States. Excerpts from them are reproduced in this chapter ("lightly" edited).* These anecdotes will, hopefully, "humanize" a little our experience in Gaza and provide some insight into the kinds of experiences you're likely to have if you participate in a program like ours. All of the persons whose anecdotes are reproduced here, incidentally, indicated that they'd welcome the opportunity to teach again in Gaza or another developing country.

****

When I arrived in Gaza, Mohammed A. was in jail. The students joked the year before that he was associated with Hamas, but nobody took it seriously until the Palestinian Authority arrested him and kept him in jail, as I recall, for nine days. Anyway he was there when we got there, and I tried to get him out by calling various places and getting enough of a positive response that an interpreter and I borrowed a car and went down to the seaside headquarters of Yasser Arafat. We were rebuffed, but the telephone calls continued and he got out. In the meantime it was a good opportunity to deliver a lecture to the class on the British tradition of habeas corpus. He told us a few things about what went on that I should not repeat but said he was instructed to say he was treated well, which he said. When I left at the end of the session, he dropped by with a couple of small gifts. He was no

---

* The anecdotes reproduced here were contributed by Dr. Kathy Chinn (University of New Mexico), Dr. Robert Moulton (University of New Mexico), Dr. Andrew Stuart (Eastern Carolina University), and Dr. Mike Zeps, S.J. (Marquette University).

terriorist, as everyone at the school agreed. [Many Palestinians, incidentally, considered members of Hamas to be freedom fighters, not terrorists.] He was outspoken and that got him in trouble; that's about it. I found him the easiest of all the students to talk with because he understood religious motivation. He even backed me up on the question of Purgatory by saying it can be found in the Koran.

****

Ziad and Abed were trained nurses before entering our program. Ziad was a family man with 6 children. He was very devoted to his wife and children. Abed was the single man when he entered our program. As we started our program, the older brother of these two had just been killed by the Israelis. Seems that as he stood next to the family barbara shop, a patrol came by and shot him (apparently for no reason) point blank in the chest. After about a year, Abed was convinced by his family to marry his dead brother's wife and take in the young child of his dead brother as his own. He did so. It was a wonderful wedding that we, as teachers, were all invited to join.

****

Reem, one of our audiology students, had a birthday party while we were there. When I walked into the party, there were only girls there (as is traditional in Arab-Islamic culture). However, none of the girls were dressed in the traditional manner with covered heads etc. Instead, they were wearing beautiful party clothes. I was walked around the circle being introduced to all the guest. What I did not know was that I was being introduced to several of my own students whom I did not recognize without their coffias (scarves). It was quite a shock.

****

The ancient Palestinian practice of arranged marriages between cousins was troubling to me. I had been taught that consanguenous marriages too often caused genetic problems (e.g., deafness and mental retardation). One of my lecture topics was the causes of deafness. Though I wasn't entirely comfortable with the decision, I did discuss the likelyhood that marriages between cousins were more likely to produce children with hearing loss than were marriages between couples who were not genetically related.

I presented the information in what I thought was a nonjudgmental way, but I must admit to hoping that the young adults in the class would be able to use the information productively, even though I knew that marriage partners were more likely to be picked by parents.

A few days after my lecture on genetics and deafness, Mona, a lovely young Bedoin student, told me that she was newly engaged. "Wonderful," I said, "tell me about the man you will marry."

I'm afraid I didn't do a good job of hiding my distress when she told me that she was engaged to her first cousin. "Don't worry," she said quickly, "he has a Ph.D. from France."

"How does his Ph.D. help with the genetic problems we talked about," I asked.

"Well," she said happily, "his Ph.D. is in genetics."

****

This story involves one of the young men in our Gazan group. Mohammed B. was an incredibly good looking fellow and so easy to like. There were no pretensions with him, nothing but a sincere desire to learn. Of all the students, he was the one to always paid close attention and, by the nature of his questions and responses, he obviously studied outside of class. He evinced some leadership, and, since he was so positive and tried so hard to do well, he was a real asset to the program.

Early on, I asked Mohammed how he got to school. He said he walked for a few miles to a main road where he caught a ride. I'm afraid that I have told similar stories about my childhood and stretched the truth a bit: "I walked to school five miles each way, uphill both ways, barefoot and without a coat, and always through deep snow, even in summer." Since I embellished, I assumed that Mohammed did, too.

I gave a midterm exam and a day or so later, before I had graded all of the tests, Mohammed asked me how he had done. He seemed quite concerned. I told him that I had not graded his exam yet, but I was sure that he had done well. "I sure hope so," he said. "I don't want to sleep with the donkey." I should have pursued this, but I let it slide.

Toward the end of program, Mohammed shyly told me that he had a new son, his first child. Not long after that, we had an evening function at school. After it ended, I caught a taxi and was riding back to my flat when I saw Mohammed walking along the side of the road. I asked the taxi driver to stop and we waited for Mohammed to catch up. I offered him a ride home but he said it would cost a lot for the taxi. "Nonsense," I said, "get in."

Mohammed gave instructions to the taxi driver who seemed quite pleased with the prospect of a relatively big fare. I guess that we drove about 15 miles before turning off the paved road. I recalled our earlier conversation and assumed, correctly, that Mohammed caught a ride at the paved road and walked the unpaved part of his daily journey to school. The dirt road was so rough that the taxi driver complained and I was afraid that I would have to experience first-hand Mohammed's daily walk. After about three miles, we arrived at a small home. Mohammed asked if I would come to see his new son and meet his family. The taxi driver agreed to wait, and I went in.

The home had three rooms and I'm sure the square footage was under 600. There was no electricity—kerosene lamps were used for light. I don't know if the house was plumbed for water or if, instead, they used an outside well. In this humble home lived Mohammed's mother and father and their twelve children. Mohammed and one brother were married and, with their wives and children, they too lived in the home.

Among other things, I wondered how Mohammed could study in this environment. I was so bold as to ask and he led me to the back of the house where a small shed housed a donkey. Next to the donkey's stall was a small table and, above it, a kerosene lamp. On the table were books relating to Mohammed's classes. Next to the table was a small bed. Mohammed explained that he studied at the table but only "slept with the donkey" when he was in trouble with his wife because of doing poorly on an examination.

****

All of the students were fantastic but Akram always stands out in my mind. He had an insatiable desire to learn about audiology. He would never leave the clinic or classroom with out being satisfied that he fully understood everything! He wanted to study and become a great clinician. When I left I knew that he would achieve his goals. I have always keep in contact with him as he wanted to know an answer to a question or requested materials for his further study. I always tried to oblige. He found employment in Gaza for several years following his graduation and then most recently was admitted to graduate school at the University of Manchester in Great Britain. I found out this past week that he had passed his exams and was one step closer toward getting his Masters degree in audiology. He once told me that I was his hero. No Akram you are my hero in showing me what dedication and determination can bring.

****

Nasser was one of the few speech-language pathology students that I had the opportunity to get to know. He was a man with many hats—friend, translator, taxi cab driver, tour guide... I always called him "The Man" and the "Treasure of Gaza." He knew everyone in Gaza both patriots and foreigners. He knew where to take to you for what ever you needed or wanted for whether it was a good meal or a relaxing glass of tea at the seashore. He always had a smile on his face and a means of making you smile. He wanted so much for Gaza to be better for his family, his people, and least of all for himself. He wanted to be the best speech-language pathology clinician. He wanted to further study abroad—a wish that was fulfilled in Great Britain. I was truly sadden the day that I heard that he had passed away while studying at the University of Lancaster. Gaza without doubt lost one of its greatest treasures the day he left us.

Sources Cited

Anderson, C. W. (1993). *Prescribing the Life of the Mind: An Essay on the Purpose of the University, the Aims of Liberal Education, the Competence of Citizens, and the Cultivation of Practical Reason.* Madison, WI: University of Wisconsin Press.

Brown, R. I., Ghazaleh, H., & Neufeldt, A. H. (1996). Challenges to rehabilitation—A case example. In Roy I. Brown, David Baine, & Aldred H. Neufeldt (Eds.), *Beyond Basic Care.* North York, Ontario, Canada: Captus Press, pp. 280-306.

Butt, G. (1995). *Life at the Crossroads: A History of Gaza.* Epping, Essex, England: Scorpion Cavendish.

Davies, R., & Johnson, P.R. (1991). *The Uzi and the Stone: Images of Gaza.* Calgary, Alberta, Canada: Detselig Enterprises Ltd.

Doughty, D., & El Aydi, M. (1995). *Gaza: A Legacy of Occupation: A Photographer's Journey.* West Hartford, CT: Kumarian Press.

Frankel, G. (1996). *Beyond the Promised Land.* New York, NY: Touchstone.

Hass, A. (1999). *Drinking the Sea at Gaza.* New York, NY: Henry Holt & Company.

Johnson, W. (1946). *People in Quandaries.* New York, NY: Harper & Brothers.

Lamb, D. (1987). *The Arabs.* New York, NY: Vintage Books.

Lederer, W. J., & Burdick, E. (1958). *The Ugly American.* New York, NY: Norton.

Qleibo, A. H. (1992). *Before the Mountains Disappear.* Kornesh EL Nill, Egypt: Al Ahram Press.

Roy, S. (1995). *Gaza Strip.* Washington, DC: Institute for Palestine Studies.

Said, E. W. (1986). *After the Last Sky: Palestinian Lives.* New York, NY: Pantheon Books.

Saunders, C. A. (1985). *A Study of the Prevalence of Handicapped Conditions Affecting Children, and a Case Finding Intervention in the Refugee Camp Population of the Gaza Strip.* Gaza: Unpublished manuscript.

Segev, T. (2000). *One Palestine, Complete: Jews and Arabs Under the British Mandate.* New York: NY: Metropolitan Books.

Silverman, F. H. (1995). *Speech, Language, and Hearing Disorders.* Boston, MA: Allyn & Bacon.

Turner, B. (Ed.) (1999). *The Statesman's Yearbook..* New York, NY: St. Martin's Press.

Index

MELLEN STUDIES IN EDUCATION

1. C. J. Schott, **Improving The Training and Evaluation of Teachers at the Secondary School Level: Educating the Educators in Pursuit of Excellence**
2. Manfred Prokop, **Learning Strategies For Second Language Users: An Analytical Appraisal with Case Studies**
3. Charles P. Nemeth, **A Status Report on Contemporary Criminal Justice Education: A Definition of the Discipline and an Assessment of Its Curricula, Faculty and Program Characteristics**
4. Stephen H. Barnes (ed.), **Points of View on American Higher Education: A Selection of Essays from *The Chronicle of Higher Education*** (Volume 1) **Professors and Scholarship**
5. Stephen H. Barnes (ed.), **Points of View on American Higher Education: A Selection of Essays from *The Chronicle of Higher Education*** (Volume 2) **Institutions and Issues**
6. Stephen H. Barnes (ed.), **Points of View on American Higher Education: A Selection of Essays from *The Chronicle of Higher Education*** (Volume 3) **Students and Standards**
7. Michael V. Belok and Thomas Metos, **The University President in Arizona 1945-1980: An Oral History**
8. Henry R. Weinstock and Charles J. Fazzaro, **Democratic Ideals and the Valuing of Knowledge In American Education: Two Contradictory Tendencies**
9. Arthur R. Crowell, Jr., **A Handbook For the Special Education Administrator: Organization and Procedures for Special Education**
10. J.J. Chambliss, **The Influence of Plato and Aristotle on John Dewey's Philosophy**
11. Alan H. Levy, **Elite Education and the Private School: Excellence and Arrogance at Phillips Exeter Academy**
12. James J. Van Patten (ed.), **Problems and Issues in College Teaching and Higher Education Leadership**
13. Célestin Freinet, **The Wisdom of Matthew: An Essay in Contemporary French Educational Theory**, John Sivell (trans.)
14. Francis R. Phillips, **Bishop Beck and English Education, 1949-1959**
15. Gerhard Falk, **The Life of the Academic Professional in America: An Inventory of Tasks, Tensions & Achievements**
16. Phillip Santa Maria, **The Question of Elementary Education in the Third Russian State Duma, 1907-1912**
17. James J. Van Patten (ed.), **The Socio-Cultural Foundations of Education and the Evolution of Education Policies in the U.S.**
18. Peter P. DeBoer, **Origins of Teacher Education at Calvin Colege, 1900-1930: And Gladly Teach**
19. Célestin Freinet, **Education Through Work: A Model for Child-Centered Learning**, John Sivell (trans.)
20. John Sivell (ed.), **Freinet Pedagogy: Theory and Practice**
21. John Klapper, **Foreign-Language Learning Through Immersion**
22. Maurice Whitehead, **The Academies of the Reverend Bartholomew Booth in Georgian England and Revolutionary America**
23. Margaret D. Tannenbaum, **Concepts and Issues in School Choice**

24. Rose M. Duhon-Sells and Emma T. Pitts, **An Interdisciplinary Approach to Multicultural Teaching and Learning**
25. Robert E. Ward, **An Encyclopedia of Irish Schools, 1500-1800**
26. David A. Brodie, **A Reference Manual for Human Performance Measurement in the Field of Physical Education and Sports Sciences**
27. Xiufeng Liu, **Mathematics and Science Curriculum Change in the People's Republic of China**
28. Judith Evans Longacre, **The History of Wilson College 1868 to 1970**
29. Thomas E. Jordan, **The First Decade of Life, Volume I: Birth to Age Five**
30. Thomas E. Jordan, **The First Decade of Life, Volume II: The Child From Five to Ten Years**
31. Mary I. Fuller and Anthony J. Rosie (eds.), **Teacher Education and School Partnerships**
32. James J. Van Patten (ed.), **Watersheds in Higher Education**
33. K. (Moti) Gokulsing and Cornel DaCosta (eds.), **Usable Knowledges as the Goal of University Education: Innovations in the Academic Enterprise Culture**
34. Georges Duquette (ed.), **Classroom Methods and Strategies for Teaching at the Secondary Level**
35. Linda A. Jackson and Michael Murray, **What Students Really Think of Professors: An Analysis of Classroom Evaluation Forms at an American University**
36. Donald H. Parkerson and Jo Ann Parkerson, **The Emergence of the Common School in the U.S. Countryside**
37. Neil R. Fenske, **A History of American Public High Schools, 1890-1990: Through the Eyes of Principals**
38. Gwendolyn M. Duhon Boudreaux (ed.), **An Interdisciplinary Approach to Issues and Practices in Teacher Education**
39. John Roach, **A Regional Study of Yorkshire Schools 1500-1820**
40. V.J. Thacker, **Using Co-operative Inquiry to Raise Awareness of the Leadership and Organizational Culture in an English Primary School**
41. Elizabeth Monk-Turner, **Community College Education and Its Impact on Socioeconomic Status Attainment**
42. George A. Churukian and Corey R. Lock (eds.), **International Narratives on Becoming a Teacher Educator: Pathways to a Profession**
43. Cecilia G. Manrique and Gabriel G. Manrique, **The Multicultural or Immigrant Faculty in American Society**
44. James J. Van Patten (ed.), **Challenges and Opportunities for Education in the 21st Century**
45. Barry W. Birnbaum, **Connecting Special Education and Technology for the 21st Century**
46. J. David Knottnerus and Frédérique Van de Poel-Knottnerus, **The Social Worlds of Male and Female Children in the Nineteenth Century French Educational System: Youth, Rituals, and Elites**
47. Sandra Frey Stegman, **Student Teaching in the Choral Classroom: An Investigation of Secondary Choral Music Student Teachers' Perceptions of Instructional Successes and Problems as They Reflect on Their Music Teaching**

48. Gwendolyn M. Duhon and Tony Manson (eds.), **Preparation, Collaboration, and Emphasis on the Family in School Counseling for the New Millennium**
49. Katherina Danko-McGhee, **The Aesthetic Preferences of Young Children**
50. Jane Davis-Seaver, **Critical Thinking in Young Children**
51. Gwendolyn M. Duhon and Tony J. Manson (eds.), **Implications for Teacher Education – Cross-Ethnic and Cross-Racial Dynamics of Instruction**
52. Samuel Mitchell, **Partnerships in Creative Activities Among Schools, Artists and Professional Organizations Promoting Arts Education**
53. Loretta Niebur, **Incorporating Assessment and the National Standards for Music Education into Everyday Teaching**
54. Tony Del Valle, **Written Literacy Features of Three Puerto Rican Family Networks in Chicago: An Ethnographic Study**
55. Christine J. Villani and Colin C. Ward, **Violence and Non-Violence in the Schools: A Manual for Administration**
56. Michael Dallaire, **Contemplation in Liberation – A Method for Spiritual Education in the Schools**
57. Gwendolyn M. Duhon, **Problems and Solutions in Urban Schools**
58. Paul Grosch, **Recognition of the Spirit and Its Development as Legitimate Concerns of Education**
59. D. Antonio Cantu, **An Investigation of the Relationship Between Social Studies Teachers' Beliefs and Practice**
60. Loretta Walton Jaggers, Nanthalia W. McJamerson and Gwendolyn M. Duhon (eds.), **Developing Literacy Skills Across the Curriculum: Practical, Approaches, Creative Models, Strategies, and Resources**
61. Haim Gordon and Rivca Gordon, **Sartre's Philosophy and the Challenge of Education**
62. Robert D. Buchanan and Ruth Ann Roberts, **Performance-Based Evaluation for Certificated and Non-Certificated School Personnel: Standards, Criteria, Indicators, Models**
63. C. David Warner III, **Opinions of Administrators, Faculty, and Students Regarding Academic Freedom and Student Artistic Expression**
64. Robert D. Heslep, **A Philosophical Guide for Decision Making by Educators: Developing a Set of Foundational Principles**
65. Noel P. Hurley, **How You Speak Determines How You Learn: Resource Allocation and Student Achievement**
66. Barry W. Birnbaum, **Foundations and Practices in the Use of Distance Education**
67. Franklin H. Silverman and Robert Moulton, **The Impact of a Unique Cooperative American University USAID Funded Speech-Language Pathologist, Audiologist, and Deaf Educator B.S. Degree Program in the Gaza Strip**